T0113411

Your
Perfectly
Pampered
Pregnancy

Beauty, Health,

and Lifestyle Advice

for the Modern

Mother-to-Be

Your Perfectly Pampered Pregnancy

Colette Bouchez

BROADWAY BOOKS
New York

Book design by Mauna Eichner

Library of Congress Cataloging-in-Publication Data

Bouchez, Colette, 1960–
    Your perfectly pampered pregnancy : beauty, health, and lifestyle advice for the modern mother-to-be / Colette Bouchez.
        p. cm.

    1. Pregnancy—Popular works. 2. Childbirth—Popular works. I. Title.
RG525.B6453 2004
618.2'4—dc21

2003049601

ISBN 978-0-7679-1442-0

146721804

Contents

Acknowledgments

I would like to express my heartfelt gratitude to the many doctors and researchers who have contributed to this book either directly through the sharing of their time, energy, and knowledge, or indirectly through their dedicated research and hard work on behalf of mothers-to-be.

I would especially like to thank the doctors and nurses of New York University Medical Center, who made invaluable contributions to this book. I am particularly indebted to Dr. Steve Goldstein, Dr. Shari Lusskin, Dr. Loren Wisner-Greene, Dr. Andrei Rebarber, Dr. Darrell Rigel, dietician and nutritionist Samantha Heller, and Dr. Gerald Verlotta, who so graciously gave me their time and never left a question unanswered. I offer a special thank-you to Dr. Jaime Grifo, director of reproductive endocrinology at New York University Medical Center, for his time and attention.

Special thanks also goes out to Dr. Charles Lockwood, chairman of obstetrics and gynecology at the Yale School of Medicine, for his invaluable research on behalf of all mothers-to-be. Thank you for always having the time to teach me something new about pregnancy. A heartfelt thank-you also belongs to Dr. Reginald Puckett of New York Presbyterian Hospital for always answering all my questions with a smile.

I am deeply grateful to Lynn Odell, vice president of public affairs for NYU Medical Center, and Nadine Woloshin of Rubinstein Associates for never failing to come up with the very best experts at all the right times.

My deepest gratitude to Greg Phillips and the staff of the American College of Obstetricians and Gynecologists, who were always there when

I needed an answer or an expert. Thank you all for always being so patient.

A salute and many thanks also goes out to my three very favorite women of style—image experts Holly Stougard-Mordini, Laura Geller, and Bobbi Brown—who so willingly passed along their secrets for helping every mother-to-be look as terrific as she feels.

My most sincere thanks goes to Broadway Books, in particular Bill Thomas, for believing that a mother-to-be is truly someone to be honored and cherished. I am grateful to senior editor Trisha Medved for her help, her inspiration, and her hard work and who, more than anyone, appreciated the reason for writing this book. And to Beth Datlowe, my heartfelt thanks for all you did every single day to keep all the wheels turning in the right direction. You are a writer's dream! And a heartfelt thank-you to Broadway deputy editorial director Stacey Creamer, for becoming the "adopted mommy" of this book, and to Sheila Klee for her keen eye and encouraging words.

A special debt of gratitude must be paid to Eleanor Rawson, the first lady of publishing, who taught me not only what it means to write a book, but what it means to be a writer. Your advice continues to echo throughout my life as it echoes throughout the pages of this book.

And what would this book be without all the great moms who helped me along the way—beginning with my own mother, who cheerfully regaled me with stories of her pregnancy with the kicking, cranky ten-month baby that I was! Special thanks also goes to Sheri, Shelly, and Nadine for letting me poke my nose into their pregnancies every chance I got. And to the dozens of mothers-to-be I met in chat rooms who so unselfishly shared their highs and lows, their questions and their woes, I am grateful to you all.

To my dear friend Tina Mosetis—thank you for all your great marketing advice and for babying the writer at the turn of every scary bend in the road. Thanks too for keeping me laughing through it all!

I must also take a moment to give a special and heartfelt thank-you to all the editors at HealthDay News Service, and The New York Times Syndicate, but in particular Jeff Walsh. You have not only shown me how good an editor can really be, but you have made me a better writer in the process—and you won't have to look hard to hear your voice throughout this book. My gratitude also goes to the editors of Web MD—thank you for making me a part of your team.

A special thank-you also goes out to Myrna Manners, Jonathan Weil, Bryan Dodson, and Kathleen Robinson of New York Presbyterian Hospital and the Weill Cornell School of Medicine and Columbia University School of Medicine, for always guiding me to the right experts. To Joanne Nicholas of Memorial Sloan-Kettering Cancer Center, a zillion thank-yous for never letting me down. And to Sandy Van and Kelli Stauning of Cedars Sinai Health System in Los Angeles goes my utmost appreciation.

And finally, my heartfelt thanks to obstetrician/gynecologist and fertility expert Dr. Niels Lauersen, a physician and healer who gave up his freedom in pursuit of better healthcare for all women. Your efforts were not in vain and your voice will never be silenced.

COLETTE BOUCHEZ

To my mother, whose infinite wisdom not only guided me through the writing of this book, but has guided me throughout my lifetime. I will be forever indebted for all you have given me and all you have done to help make my dreams come true. And to my dad, whose memory is with me every single day and who, to this day, reminds me I am never alone.

To St. Jude, truly the patron saint of writers: I will be forever grateful for all the blessings you have brought into my life.

To Julia Hannah, Brooke Allison, and Darcie, the Princess of Pinkland—three little girls who personify the strength to which all big girls aspire.

And for David . . . the sound of your laughter still melts my heart.

Introduction

Who's That Girl in the "Pregnant" Mirror?

I've always believed that one of the truly wonderful things about women is our instinctual ability to nurture and care for those we love. From our mates to our children, our family to our friends, there is no question that we are blessed with a very unique ability to make those we love feel cared for and cherished. Never are these warm, nurturing, *motherly* instincts more powerful or in sharper focus than during pregnancy—a time when our body, mind, and spirit become enraptured with bringing that precious new life into the world.

But as we concentrate on doing *everything* right for our baby, too often, it seems, we can begin to lose sight of ourselves. As we continue to put our own needs on the back burner while still giving 110 percent to our family, our job, and especially the brand-new life growing inside us, it's not uncommon to one day find ourselves gazing at our own image and wondering: Who *is* that girl in the pregnant mirror? Everything about the way we look and feel has seemed to change.

And while most of us are prepared for the big differences—the ever-growing tummy and even the weight gain—what can take many of us by surprise is the way all the little pieces in our lives no longer seem to fit in quite the same way. Having a baby, it seems, not only affects how we physically look and feel, but it also influences how we think and act and react to everything in our world.

Will you be deliriously happy? At times you will be *so happy* you can hardly believe how great you feel. You will find overwhelming new joy in the simplest of life's pleasures—like listening to the beating of your baby's heart or feeling those glorious kicks of life inside you for the very first time. And as you pat your growing tummy falling asleep at night, you'll know the wondrous new feeling that you will never again be alone in the world—that you are a part of someone and they a part of you forever.

But just as many times you will feel the bumps in the road—the lows, the self-doubts, the fears, and the anxieties that can, at times, seem overwhelming. If your pregnancy was unexpected and not an event you anticipated or planned, you may even be plagued with feelings of resentment or anger—emotions you can find hard to reconcile with your new-found feelings of joy.

But whether or not your baby was planned, pregnancy may still find you viewing every facet of your life under a microscope, continually re-examining how you feel about your baby, your partner, your career, even your relationship to your own mother. Will I be a good parent? What's going to happen to my career? How is my marriage going to change? Will I be able to manage everything? Your mind doesn't stop racing. In fact, what seemed like such a simple idea just a few months ago—becoming a mother—may now seem like an *enormous* task, one that is threatening to swallow you whole.

If, in fact, this *is* how you sometimes feel, it's important to realize you are not alone. An overwhelming majority of women share at least some of your concerns, worries, and fears. What can help you find your way out of the forest? Learning how to free up and refocus at least some of those energies so that you can concentrate just a little bit more on *you.* And that is precisely the philosophy behind *Your Perfectly Pampered Pregnancy,* a brand-new kind of guide dedicated solely to helping you care for yourself while you care for your baby.

Certainly, the health and welfare of your unborn child is and will remain the focal point of your life in the coming months. And it remains of tantamount importance to continue to do everything you can to ensure that your baby will come into the world as perfect as he or she can be. But equally important is that you also come to recognize and honor your own needs—both physical and emotional—and not lose sight of who you are as you travel the road to motherhood.

Your New Pregnant Life: What to Expect

Chances are you've already had one or more prenatal visits to your obstetrician. If so, then you may also know that the time you will spend with your doctor is never nearly enough. And because all attention is on baby—including that of your physician—you may even feel that the questions you have about yourself are not only going unanswered, in many instances they aren't even being heard.

The good news: *Your Perfectly Pampered Pregnancy* throws open the doors to a plethora of answers concerning the ways in which your pregnancy is affecting you—from head to toe. It all begins, in Chapter 1, with a look at your physical health during pregnancy and what you can expect from your body, from first trimester to last. From morning sickness to stretch marks, hemorrhoids to varicose veins, vaginal infections to backaches, heartburn, and more, you'll find the explanations and the solutions for the most common health concerns likely to *invade* your life sometime over the next eight or nine months. Moving on to slightly more serious problems, you'll also find a primer on high blood pressure in pregnancy and some of its more complex consequences. You'll not only learn how to know if you are at risk, but the steps your doctor must take in order to protect your health. Likewise you'll find the newest data available on gestational diabetes, including how to protect yourself and your baby should pregnancy cause your sugar levels to rise.

Chapter 2 provides important advice and information on your intimate anatomy—beginning with a comprehensive new look at your pregnant V zone, that ultra-special area between your growing belly and your thighs. You'll learn how your intimate anatomy changes during pregnancy and how to adjust your personal hygiene routines accordingly, plus how to recognize the signs of V zone trouble. You'll even discover what you can do right now to begin conditioning your pelvic and vaginal muscles for childbirth, making labor and delivery safer *and* easier for you and your baby. There's an entire section devoted to your breast health during pregnancy and special advice on why you don't have to worry about the lumps and bumps that can develop during this special time. You'll also learn how to do a pregnancy breast self-exam and discover why you must never skip this vital opportunity for self-care.

In Chapter 3 you're invited to a comprehensive crash course in some of the changes you'll see when you gaze into that "pregnant" mirror for the very first time—changes in your skin, including not only your face, but your overall body complexion. While some of the information you'll find here is good common sense that works equally well whether you're pregnant or not, much of it is specific to the skin you're in right now. The pregnancy mask, stretch marks, simple rashes, and complex dermatological conditions—they're all covered with advice from some of the nation's leading dermatologists and obstetricians.

You've Got Style!

Shifting gears once again, Chapter 4 helps you explore and find your personal pregnancy style—the "you" the rest of the world sees during each of your trimesters. With special advice on fashion, hair, and makeup, you'll be treated to tips and tricks from some of the world's top style experts—including makeup artists Laura Geller, Bobbi Brown, and Holly Stougard-Mordini—the very same experts who regularly help some of Hollywood's top celebrities look *their* best. You'll even get advice from some celebrity moms on how to pamper your body, mind, and spirit Hollywood style.

In addition, there are some fun and interesting facts about how to find the best pregnancy undergarments, from panties to bras, girdles to hose, plus the least expensive ways to put together a super maternity work wardrobe, including how to find the best fashion bargains no matter where you live. But the style advice doesn't stop here. While many of you will find that pregnancy is just three glorious trimesters of great hair days, for those who don't there's a bonnetful of advice on everything from styling aids and shampoos to coloring and perming products—you'll even learn how to make all-natural hair styling products that baby your hair while you protect your baby.

Next it's on to your diet and fitness needs. Chapters 5 and 6 are jam-packed with the latest information on the foods, vitamins, and fitness workouts that can help you remain healthy and strong throughout your pregnancy and beyond. You'll learn how to adapt baby-friendly nutrients to an adult-friendly palate, how to nutritiously cope with food aversions and cravings, and how to find the foods that satisfy your hunger without toppling your pregnancy scale. You'll even discover how to test your prenatal vitamin to ensure you're getting all the nutrients you really need. Plus, you'll not only discover the most effective workouts for a faster, easier labor, but you'll learn what you can do *during* your pregnancy to make weight loss faster and easier *after* you give birth. Even more important: Being pregnant no longer means having to give up your favorite sporting activities. A new guide shows you how to modify even the most adventurous activities so that now nearly anything you enjoy doing can be made pregnancy-friendly and baby-safe.

Stress, Sex, and Pregnancy

From the ring of our cell phone to the buzz of our beeper to the honk of the horn from the car behind us, pregnant or not, there's no hiding from stress. What's more, studies show that you may be even more vulnerable to the effects of stress when you are pregnant—one more good reason to be extra vigilant when caring for yourself and your needs. In eye-opening Chapter 7 you'll learn all the ways that stress can secretly affect your pregnant body—sometimes without your even realizing what's going on—and how you can counter the effects and emerge stronger and healthier than ever. If you must endure a personal tragedy while you are pregnant, you'll learn the steps to immediately take to protect yourself and your baby from harm. You'll also find some fun and practical ways to turn down the volume of stress in your life via activities like partner massage and aromatherapy. You'll even discover how to indulge your relaxation fantasies with a pregnancy spa bath designed to tickle your senses as it relaxes your body and your mind.

Moving on, what pregnancy would be complete without at least a few problems with S-E-X? In fact, no matter how many glorious stories you've heard about how terrific your pregnant sex life can be (and it can!), what your friends might not be so quick to divulge is how many problems can get in the way of your bliss. In Chapter 8 you'll find the kinds of situations and conditions that can frequently come between you and your partner—including eight common fears about making pregnant love—plus the solutions that can help. You'll learn how to stay close to your partner, even when intercourse is not possible, and when it is, you'll discover the safest ways to have sex—including the six best and most comfortable positions for you and your partner. You'll even learn some important news about how your own sex drive may change during your pregnancy and how to bring the romance back into your life after your baby is born.

Pregnancy and the World Around You

Those of you who plan to work through your pregnancy and continue to push forward on your career goals won't want to skip Chapter 9. Here you'll find not only some of the best practical *and* legal advice for ensuring that your workplace is a safe place for you and your baby, you'll also discover important ways to work with your doctor to help ensure your health through all nine working months.

Perhaps even more important, you'll find some new insights on the social interplay that can occur between you and your coworkers while you are pregnant, with advice concerning the best and most professional ways to announce your pregnancy. You'll even learn how to deal with everything from coworkers who ignore your condition, to those who want to know way too much information, to a boss who may be less than thrilled with your news.

Chapter 10 provides calming and reassuring advice on the best ways to cope with the lifestyle issues that are undoubtedly part of your world. Is it okay to use a cell phone? Can I work on my computer? Is it safe to varnish my floors or paint the nursery? What about West Nile virus and the smallpox vaccine: What do I need to know? You'll find the answers to these and dozens more questions, along with the latest facts on smoking, alcohol, caffeine, and other factors that might affect you while you are pregnant.

And because virtually every pregnancy spans the better part of a year, this book would not be complete without Chapter 11, dedicated to year-round pregnancy care. From summer allergies to winter colds, chronic migraines to asthma events, you'll find helpful and reassuring information on the best and safest ways to care for yourself through all nine months, no matter when in the year your pregnancy occurs.

Bathing in the Afterglow

As your pregnancy winds down and the excitement of your delivery date draws near, I can promise you that even the very worst days of each trimester will be nothing more than a fading memory. But as you approach the next phase of your life—as a new mom—you should not abandon your need for some serious TLC. In fact, if you promise that you won't skimp on self-care in the days and weeks following the birth of your baby, I can promise you a faster and easier recovery—and a good chance that you can protect yourself from the ravages of some serious postpartum problems.

In this final chapter you will find all the basics to pull you through the first six hours, six days, and six weeks after giving birth. From what to expect from your body to how you will feel emotionally, how to know when it's safe to begin exercising, how long it will take to lose your "baby fat," when your sex life will return and when to return to work—here you'll find the quintessential summary of the most important information you need to go forward into motherhood. In a very vital and poignant section you'll find understanding and compassionate advice on how to cope with the "baby blues," including when it's time to talk to your doctor about how you feel.

Finally, you'll discover an extraordinary Resource Center with information on every self-care product and service discussed in this book, as well as the medical experts and medical journals consulted throughout. You'll even find a listing of the government agencies and medical organizations that can cut through the red tape and help you get additional facts and information to take care of all your pregnancy needs.

Your Perfectly Pampered Pregnancy is your ultimate pregnancy self-care guide—a book that will lovingly lead you from your first trimester through to your delivery day and beyond, with information and solutions, understanding and compassion, and the kind of tender loving care that, ultimately, will help you have not only a happier, more peaceful, more stress-free pregnancy but, in the end, a healthier baby.

Most important, however, I hope you will come to see that *Your Perfectly Pampered Pregnancy* is more than just a collection of facts and information—it is a philosophy, and one that I hope you will embrace now and for the rest of your life. My message: The importance of recognizing your own needs and remembering to care for yourself, even when the demands on your time and your energy and your heart may threaten to cloud the vision of who you really are and what you need.

Indeed, as you go forward into your pregnancy, remember that giving life to that wonderful little person growing inside you doesn't have to mean losing the person who you are. The baby you are creating isn't taking *your* life away—rather it is *your life* that is making this brand-new baby possible. So be kind to yourself, stay in touch with who you are, and treat yourself with the loving care and respect that you deserve. That is the philosophy of *Your Perfectly Pampered Pregnancy.*

Thank you for making me a part of your pregnancy. I wish good health and happiness for you and your baby, and may the days that lie ahead be the best you have ever known.

If I can ever help you or answer any of your questions, please don't hesitate to write me. Also remember to visit my website—www.pamper ingmom.com—where you'll find the very latest information to help make your pregnancy as happy and as healthy as it can be.

My best regards—and congratulations.

COLETTE BOUCHEZ
DearColette@Pamperingmom.com

Oh! My Aching Pregnancy

Solutions for Your Most Common
Health Problems

Whether you've just discovered you're pregnant, or you've known for a while that baby is on the way, chances are you have already begun to notice changes in your body. The most obvious, of course, will be in your breasts and particularly your tummy, both of which will take on a totally new shape and feel. As your uterus stretches to make room for your growing baby, and your breasts begin developing the milk ducts that will nourish and feed your newborn, your pregnancy clearly begins to "show." The closer you get to your delivery date, the more your "state of grace" will become obvious, not only to you but to the world around you.

But long before that happens, there are a series of *other* changes that will take place as well. Most, if not all, will stem from the sudden increase in estrogen and progesterone—the hormones of pregnancy that began coursing through your body from almost the moment you conceived.

For most of you, these sometimes dramatic and definitely abrupt changes will affect the way you feel, both physically and emotionally, often right from the start of your pregnancy. Morning sickness, fatigue, mood swings—these are just some of the problems that may seem to rob you of at least some of the joy you initially felt when you learned you were pregnant.

As you go forward with your pregnancy, you may be focusing your attention on even more significant concerns, such as the risk of high blood pressure, preeclampsia, or high blood sugar—all real and frightening conditions that threaten not only your pregnancy but your personal health as well.

The important thing to remember, however, is that for the most part, nearly *everything* you will experience is a normal and natural part of your pregnancy. What's more, most of these problems will gently pass as you move from one trimester to the next. And while each one may get you down for a little while, with a little bit of knowledge and some generous self-care, you can not only quickly resolve many of the problems you will experience, but in some instances, even learn how to prevent some from occurring at all.

As a result, your journey into motherhood will begin with a new confidence—a state of mind that will not only help you to weather all the bumps in the road but to do so with infinitely more style and grace.

Before you begin to explore the various problems that *might* occur—and the solutions that can help—it's important to remember that no two pregnancies run on the exact same timetable. So, while many of the conditions mentioned in this chapter are rooted in specific trimesters, don't be alarmed if what you experience occurs earlier or later, lasts longer or stops sooner, or doesn't occur at all!

It's also important that you always check any *new* symptoms with your doctor, even if you're certain you know what's wrong. Chances are, whatever you experience will be a normal and predictable part of pregnancy. But only your doctor can know for certain—so don't skip getting his or her expert opinion on whatever problems come your way.

The Five Most Common Pregnancy
Complaints and How to Fix Them

PROBLEM #1: MORNING SICKNESS

Ever since that day in the 1950s when a blossoming and pregnant Lucy Ricardo announced to the television world that she was "nauseous," morning sickness came bounding out of the closet and into our everyday pregnancy vocabulary. But perhaps the greatest misconception about this common pregnancy concern is that it occurs *only* in the morning. In truth, the nausea and vomiting that are the hallmarks of this condition can actually occur *any time* of the day or night. It is often prompted by the smell or taste of certain foods, and usually occurs within the first four to eight weeks of pregnancy. It has, however, been known to develop as soon as fourteen days after conception.

For some women, the symptoms can continue to build until about the fourteenth or even the sixteenth week, after which they rapidly disappear. For most, however, morning sickness *gradually* subsides so that by week thirteen or fourteen, you are feeling substantially better, with nearly all symptoms gone. In the meantime, the degree to which you experience morning sickness can range from mild queasiness to frequent vomiting or anything in between. Fatigue and headaches are also commonly part of the picture. The important thing to remember is that, in general, morning sickness is a common part of pregnancy and so long as it remains within the normal time frame, it's not considered harmful to you or baby.

WHY MORNING SICKNESS OCCURS

While no one is certain exactly why morning sickness occurs, most experts believe that the pregnancy hormone hCG—short for human chorionic gonadotropin—plays a big role. Perhaps not coincidentally, levels of hCG are highest during the first trimester, when the risk of morning sickness is greatest. "Levels also soar in mothers of twins and triplets, which is also the group most likely to suffer the most severe morning sickness," says Dr. Steve Goldstein, professor of obstetrics and gynecology at New York University School of Medicine.

Studies show problems can also develop as a result of the quick rise in estrogen and progesterone that occurs in early pregnancy. As levels of these hormones climb, they can temporarily change the muscle contractions and relaxation patterns of your stomach and intestines, which further increases feelings of nausea.

A controversial new theory says morning sickness may be nature's way of protecting a pregnancy. Cornell researchers Samuel Flaxman and Paul Sherman report that the foods which most commonly trigger pregnancy nausea—meat, fish, and poultry—were once considered to carry the highest rate of foodborne pathogens—bacteria that could increase the risk of miscarriage. Nausea in the presence of these foods may have been nature's way of keeping mothers-to-be from eating potentially harmful foods, says Flaxman. Oddly enough, these researchers found that women who experienced the *most* nausea and vomiting during pregnancy are the least likely to suffer a miscarriage. A similar theory published in the *Journal of Obstetrics and Gynecology* in May 2000 says that morning sickness may promote a healthy pregnancy by controlling the production of insulin and other hormones that could interfere with the growth of the placenta, the protective sac of fluids and nutrients that surrounds your baby in the womb.

So, while it may leave you feeling less than great, take comfort in knowing that morning sickness can be the sign of a healthy pregnancy. Of course, that doesn't mean you won't want to control symptoms or, if possible, make them disappear. To this end, experts from the Mayo Clinic, along with members of the American College of Obstetricians and Gynecologists, have devised a series of survival tips—advice that may help pull you through a few dreadful morning (or evening) moments. While some of these suggestions are based on common sense and well-worn pieces of advice, others may provide you with new and surprisingly practical options.

SURVIVING MORNING SICKNESS: ONE DOZEN THINGS YOU CAN TRY RIGHT NOW

1. *Identify Personal Nausea Triggers.* While in the beginning it may seem as if *everything makes you nauseous,* in reality, most women re-

spond to just a few external cues. In addition to the smell of meat, fish, and poultry, other common odor triggers include greasy, fatty foods, coffee, onions, garlic, and pungent spices. In a medical report published in the October 2000 issue of the journal *Female Patient,* researchers say even environmental factors can be a trigger, particularly cleaning or workplace chemicals, perfume, heat, humidity, noise, motion (like riding in an elevator or on a subway), or even a flickering computer screen. By identifying your nausea triggers, you can work on reducing exposure—which in turn can dramatically or even completely eliminate episodes of morning sickness.

2. *Mommy Want a Cracker?* Eat a dry, high-carbohydrate snack, such as crackers or toast, *twenty to thirty minutes before* you get out of bed in the morning, and avoid drinking any liquids, particularly water, during this time. Doing so can calm the queasies before they start and get your day off on the right foot.

3. *Never Go to Bed Hungry.* Since low blood sugar can sometimes trigger nausea, eat a high-protein snack, such as cheese or egg salad, before bedtime. Also avoid high-sugar snacks or simple carbohydrates late at night, since they can cause a drop in blood sugar and precipitate morning nausea.

4. *Limit Fluid Intake with Meals.* Instead, drink between meals, and try tummy-soothing beverages like ginger tea, ginger ale, or decaffeinated black or green tea.

5. *Switch Prenatal Vitamins or the Time You Take Them.* The high iron content in most prenatal vitamins can leave you feeling nauseous much of the time. So, talk to your doctor about switching to a low-iron or even no-iron formula for the first trimester, when the risk of anemia, and your need for iron, is lowest. Sometimes just switching brands can also make a difference, even if the iron content stays the same. In addition, you can try taking your vitamins late in the day, and instead of swallowing the pills with water, try putting them in a spoonful of pudding or applesauce.

6. *Try the BRATT Diet.* Short for bananas, rice, applesauce, toast, and tea. Many experts say these foods may help calm a queasy stomach, reduce intestinal contractions, and help control vomiting.

7. *Eat or Drink Anything Containing Ginger.* It's not just an old wives' tale! Studies published in the April 2001 issue of the journal *Obstetrics and Gynecology* show that ginger really does control the nausea and vomiting of pregnancy. In a survey conducted by the American College of Obstetricians and Gynecologists, some 52 percent of all obstetricians now recommend ginger for pregnancy patients. While natural ginger is best, as a tea or sprinkled over a dessert, you can also try drinking ginger ale or eating ginger snaps, or talk to your doctor about taking ginger capsules. If you don't like the taste or smell of ginger, try anything lemon flavored (hard candy, sorbet, lemonade) or peppermint gum or candy. Be aware, however, that peppermint may increase your risk of heartburn, so don't take it after a meal. For a quick fix away from home try Preggie Pops—all-natural lollipops in flavors like ginger, lavender, mint, and sour fruits, which studies show can help reduce nausea.

8. *Massage Your Pressure Points.* Putting pressure on what Chinese medicine experts call the P6 Nei Guan nerve located in the wrist can calm a queasy stomach almost immediately. You can stimulate this nerve, located on the underside of the arm about two inches above the wrist, with pressure from two fingers or the thumb of your opposite hand. You can also invest in an acupressure band— a bracelet worn around the wrist that continually stimulates the antinausea point. Sold in drugstores as a motion sickness treat- ment, or under the name Relief Bands, in one medical study, 70 percent of the pregnant women who wore these wristbands found immediate relief.

9. *Turn Down the Lights—and the Stress.* For many women, morn- ing sickness fades in a dimly lit and quiet environment—which, not surprisingly, is often the hospital treatment for severe nausea. Turn lights low, crack a window for fresh air and circulation, and place a rolled towel at the base of your bedroom door to keep out

any offensive odors from kitchen or bath. According to Dr. John Larsen, chairman of maternal-fetal medicine at George Washington University, stress can also make vomiting worse, so try to eliminate as much tension from your life as you can. In addition, remember that fatigue can encourage morning sickness, so don't overlook the power of a nap to reduce that nauseous feeling.

10. *Rise and Shine . . . Slowly.* When you do get up—whether in the morning or after a nap—do so slowly. Rising too quickly can throw off your equilibrium and contribute to the queasies.

11. *Eat Often.* Instead of three meals a day, opt for six smaller ones. If your nausea is particularly severe, Brigham and Women's Hospital dietician Miriam Erick advises you to eat whatever you can, whenever you can—calories in any form will sustain you until nausea passes.

12. *Stick It to Morning Sickness.* The treatment is acupuncture, a procedure that uses a series of needles painlessly placed just below the surface of the skin—in this case, just above the wrist—in order to stimulate nerve endings linked to nausea. Studies published in the American journal *Birth* in February 2002 found that just four weekly twenty-minute acupuncture treatments dramatically reduced nausea and vomiting in some 600 women. For many, relief was seen in just one treatment. These findings echoed an earlier study in 2000 that found acupuncture reduced nausea in more than half of the pregnant women in the group. **One caveat:** Make certain that you choose a licensed acupuncturist, and that he or she uses only disposable needles (to reduce the risk of infection). Also, get the okay of your obstetrician or midwife *before* getting treatment.

The Smell of Success:
How Aromatherapy Can Help You

Although for most women smells and aromas can be a leading trigger for bouts of morning sickness, a few scents may actually help you to overcome your nausea. Based on principles of aromatherapy—that certain scents have the ability to trigger complex neurological reactions—the key here is to use *essential oils* that have been shown to calm areas of the brain linked to the nausea response. While many women find that certain scents can relieve their nauseous feelings, it's a good idea to take your first sniff when you aren't feeling queasy—just to make certain the oils don't irritate your sinuses or bring on any allergies. That said, here are a few classic recipes you can try.

Morning Sickness Remedy
To a bowl of water, add 3 drops of lavender oil and 1 drop of peppermint oil. Stir and inhale. You can also try a cool compress soaked in a lavender solution on your forehead or a warm lavender compress on your chest. For many women, a sniff of peppermint oil is all that's necessary to head off a bout of pregnancy nausea. For others, peppermint enhances the aromas of certain foods and actually increases nausea. But even if you find that peppermint does help you, **never** use a highly concentrated oil preparation, internally or externally, particularly during your first trimester. Some herbalists believe that because peppermint has a stimulating effect, it can, at least theoretically, stimulate uterine contractions and increase your risk of miscarriage. In addition, when taken on an empty stomach, even small concentrations of peppermint may increase your risk of heartburn and gastrointestinal distress during pregnancy.

Instant Antinausea Remedy
To combat any offensive odors you may encounter outside your home, aromatherapy expert Marlene Ericksen suggests dousing a hankie with a light peppermint/lavender blend and keeping it in a sealed plastic bag inside your handbag. At the first hint of nausea, hold the hankie over your nose and inhale once or twice.

When Morning Sickness Won't Go Away: What to Do

For most women, morning sickness begins to disappear by the third month of pregnancy, or sometimes even before. Some, however, are not quite so lucky. Each year some 55,000 pregnant women are hospitalized for hyperemesis gravidarium—morning sickness that just won't quit. For these women, holding down any food becomes increasingly impossible, while constant vomiting results in weight loss, dehydration, and an imbalance of key nutrients like sodium and potassium. If not treated, problems may progress to include neurological disturbances and, in severe cases, even liver damage and death.

While no one is certain why this condition occurs, early research points to exceedingly high estrogen levels as one source of the problem. According to Dr. Andrei Rebarber, director of maternal-fetal medicine at New York University Medical Center, the problem may also be related to higher than normal levels of the hormone hCG or to certain placenta-related conditions.

According to researcher Lisa Signorello, high fat consumption before or during pregnancy may also be linked to severe morning sickness. In her study, published in the November 1998 issue of the journal *Epidemiology*, women who ate 30 grams of saturated fat daily (equal to about two quarter-pound cheeseburgers) were five times more likely to develop this problem than those who consumed just 15 grams of fat a day. Again, the link is estrogen, since, says Signorello, women who eat high levels of saturated fat generally make more estrogen. So, while consuming less saturated fat may help, remember that sometimes even pregnant vegetarians or athletes develop this problem.

The important thing to remember is that with treatment, women with even the most severe cases of hyperemesis gravidarium recover and have healthy babies. The key is alerting your doctor as soon as nausea, and particularly vomiting, gets out of hand. Don't wait until the nausea becomes unbearable, advises Dr. Rebarber, since there are a number of safe medications that can help. Among the most popular treatments, he says, is a combination of the over-the-counter sleep aid Unisom in conjunction with 50 milligrams of vitamin B_6 daily, both of which have been proven safe for both mom and baby. Although both medications are available without a prescription, **never take this or any combination without checking with your doctor first.**

Other drugs that can help include the medication Reglan (metoclopromide), which works by increasing the rate at which the stomach and intestines move during digestion and by increasing the speed at which the stomach empties. Both factors can work to control the nausea and vomiting of pregnancy. Recently Reglan has become available as an infusion pump, which allows you to receive the medication even if you are unable to swallow or hold down the tablets.

For some women, antihistamines, including the allergy medication Benadryl (diphenhydramine) or the classic seasickness remedy Dramamine (dimenydrinate), can help. Again, however, **never use any medication to treat your morning sickness on your own.** While these treatments are safe to use, says Dr. Rebarber, the exact dosage will depend on many factors linked to *your* personal pregnancy—and only your doctor can tell you how much to take and how often. If you are throwing up more than twice a day or are unable to keep any food or liquid down, call your doctor as soon as possible and seek treatment.

PROBLEM #2: BACKACHE

Just as the nausea of your first trimester winds down, you may find it is replaced with another pregnancy problem: backaches. Affecting some 50 percent of all pregnant women, symptoms often begin around the sixth month and, for some, can continue up to six months after giving birth. If you suffered with back problems prior to getting pregnant, your risk is higher once you conceive.

According to a Swedish study published in the journal *Spine* in 1991, most pregnancy backaches occur in either the lumbar area (between the waist and the shoulder blades) or in the sacroiliac area (several inches below the waist). But Denver orthopedist Dr. Julie Colliton reports that many women also experience pain in the lower half of their buttocks, radiating down all or part of their leg. In a paper published in the July 1996 issue of the journal *The Physician and Sports Medicine,* she points out that while many women feel the most pain when running or walking up or down stairs, don't be surprised if you also feel discomfort with simple movements, like turning over in bed, getting in and out of your car, or lifting or twisting. You may even find that sitting or standing for long periods of time without changing position can cause back problems. A condition known as nocturnal back pain can cause discomfort as soon as you lie down.

WHAT CAUSES PREGNANCY BACKACHES

Regardless of the type of pain you experience, experts say the cause is nearly always rooted in biomechanical and physiological changes that begin in the second trimester. As your uterus rapidly expands, your entire spine shifts backward, along with your center of gravity. This, in turn, throws off your balance. As your body tries to compensate for the changes, you make subtle shifts in posture that ultimately can put significant stress on your back.

In addition, your body is also producing the hormone relaxin, which increases joint laxity so delivery is easier. In the meantime, however, it temporarily weakens the support system in the joints of your lower back, which can result in increased pain when walking or standing. Many doctors also believe that relaxin may increase your risk of back injury by loosening ligaments and joints in the pelvis, which in turn increases the risk of sprains, particularly when lifting. You can prevent many backaches and back injuries by making sure you always bend your knees before lifting and confine what you do lift to lighter loads. (See "Squat" on page 12.) General rule of thumb: If you have to strain to pick it up, don't pick it up.

If you have already begun to experience backache, there are steps you can take to help diminish your pain. If pain has not yet started, in many instances these same steps can help prevent back pain from ever occurring. To help get you started, experts from the American College of Obstetricians and Gynecologists offer the following suggestions.

TEN WAYS TO REDUCE PREGNANCY
BACK PAIN NATURALLY

1. Exercise, Exercise, Exercise!
If you start the back-strengthening workouts featured in Chapter 5 before your pain begins, you may head off the risk of problems and avoid many back complaints. If pain has already started, these same simple moves can help realign your spine and reduce pressure, helping to keep backaches in check. What can also help: maintaining proper posture, not only when you stand, but also when you sit. Making a conscious effort to sit as straight as possible can help create the posture mind-set that will carry over when you stand or walk.

2. Go Shoe Shopping

If you have a passion for buying shoes—lucky you—pregnancy gives you a great excuse for a whole new footwear wardrobe. Surprisingly, the best shoes to reduce backaches are not flats or even sneakers. They can shift your gravity center even farther out of alignment. Instead, experts say to look for low-heeled shoes—about 1.5 to 2 inches in height—with good arch supports. If you love the shoes but support is minimal, invest in an orthotic—a removable arch support you can change from shoe to shoe. Another reason to shoe-shop during pregnancy: Your foot size may increase. Since nerve endings in feet are ultra-sensitive, wearing shoes that are too tight or too short may contribute to back or leg pain.

3. Get on Your Soap Box

And use it to elevate one foot whenever you must stand for any significant length of time. By bending your knee and keeping your foot propped 6 to 8 inches off the ground, you can dramatically reduce back pressure and keep muscles from tensing and cramping.

4. Get a Board in Bed

Slipped under your mattress, a bed board can increase the support of your sleep surface, which in turn may reduce back pain. This is particularly important if pregnancy weight is causing you to sleep in a gully of indented space. The board will add the additional support you need and help keep your spine straight—but remember, you want to sleep on your left side, not your back, to help increase circulation and speed the flow of nutrients to your baby.

5. Squat

As unpleasant as it sounds, squatting rather than bending from the waist to pick up *anything* can go a long way in preventing muscle twists and turns that increase back pain. Remember to keep your back straight and lower your body slowly—and never pick up anything that stresses your muscles. If you already have one or more children who are used to having Mom lift and carry, ask your partner to step in and tote those toddlers for a while.

6. Carry a Pillow Everywhere

Using a small cushion to support your lower back can do wonders for re-ducing back strain. Take it everywhere—on the bus, in the car, to your job, to the pizza place—whenever you're going to sit for more than ten minutes.

7. More Pillow Talk

This time, tuck the pillow between your knees when lying on your side. It will help remove pressure from your spine, and you're likely to feel im-mediate relief. If you don't, add a second pillow.

8. Get in on Girdle Power

A pregnancy girdle—one specially constructed to support your back without compromising circulation to your tummy—can dramatically re-duce back pain. You can also try a traditional pregnancy tummy sling—a band that runs from two points on the center of your back, down under your stomach, to support your tummy, pelvis, uterus, plus your baby and your back. See Chapter 4 for more information on what to look for in a pregnancy girdle.

9. Heat, Cold, Massage

Hot or cold compresses, alone or in combination with massage, can be major pain relievers. While heat can add comfort, cold will numb pain, and massage can work the knots out of sore tired muscles and increase cir-culation—which may also rejuvenate slightly injured muscles. See Chap-ter 7 for the best pregnancy backrub techniques.

10. Get Connected

If back pain becomes overwhelming, talk to your doctor about TENS ther-apy—short for transcutaneous electrical nerve stimulation. Here a thera-pist attaches small lead wires to the surface of your skin and then sends harmless electrical impulses to muscles and nerves for twenty to forty min-utes. The result can be immediate pain relief that lasts. While studies show that TENS is safe for most women to use during pregnancy, make sure to discuss it with your obstetrician first. Doctors say back treatments to *avoid* during pregnancy include whirlpool therapy or joint manipulation.

PROBLEM #3: HEARTBURN AND
GASTROINTESTINAL UPSETS

If you're like most women, the one pregnancy problem you probably won't escape is heartburn. Occurring during any of your trimesters and sometimes lasting clear through to delivery, you may be constantly or intermittently plagued with not only heartburn, but burping, indigestion, even pain in your esophagus.

The problem is once again those pregnancy hormones, which slow digestion, leaving food in your stomach longer. This, in turn, increases the risk that acid will splash into your esophagus and ignite the burn. In addition, high levels of the hormone progesterone can also cause the muscle between your esophagus and stomach to relax, making it easier for this to occur. If your heartburn begins or worsens in your third trimester, your growing uterus is likely to blame. As your baby enlarges, your uterus pushes upward into your stomach, bringing the contents closer to your esophagus and making it much easier for acids to backwash and cause problems.

COPING WITH HEARTBURN: WHAT TO TRY

Most doctors agree that your first line of defense is to avoid large meals and spicy foods—both of which can encourage more acid production. Additionally, if you prevent your stomach from being totally empty, you may find you have less heartburn, since the gastric juices associated with hunger can contribute to the discomfort. If you have not stopped smoking, now is the time to do so, since this too can contribute to your heartburn.

If your gastric problems occur mostly at night, watch your bedtime snacks, avoiding spicy or fatty foods as well as caffeine, chocolate, and carbonated beverages. To further reduce risks, chew gum after each meal—but don't select a mint variety. Although peppermints are the classic after-dinner treat, studies show that when taken after a meal, mint relaxes the muscle between the esophagus and stomach. This allows acids in your stomach to more easily reach your esophagus, thus *increasing* your risk of heartburn.

Finally, you can also try raising the head of your bed, either by plac-

Real Life

UNDERSTANDING YOUR PREGNANCY PAINS

Q: I've just started my second trimester and I've begun to get some sharp pains in my abdomen, going down into my groin. I was afraid at one point I was getting a hernia. Is this anything to worry about, and should I talk to my doctor?

A: First, always discuss any pain you feel during pregnancy with your doctor—if for no other reason than to ease your mind. That said, according to experts at the Mayo Clinic, abdominal pain during the second trimester is often related to the stretching of the muscles and ligaments surrounding your expanding uterus. A sudden movement or even a long stretch or reach can tug on the round cordlike ligament that supports your uterus, resulting in a pulling or even a stabbing pain in your lower pelvis or groin. Some women even experience a sharp pain in their side—almost like a "stitch" you get from running.

Additionally, previous abdominal surgery, including fertility procedures, can result in adhesions or scar tissue—bands of fibrous tissue that form in and around your uterus. As your baby grows, the bands can stretch or pull apart, also resulting in pain.

Regardless of the cause, whatever pain you feel should stop within a few minutes. If it doesn't, particularly if it continues more than twenty or thirty minutes, or if it grows worse in intensity, call your doctor right away.

ing blocks under the legs supporting your headboard or by using a foam sleeping wedge that elevates your upper body.

HEARTBURN TREATMENTS:
HOW YOUR DOCTOR CAN HELP

For many doctors, the first line of defense *after dietary modifications* is simple antacids—drugs like Tums, Pepcid AC, Mylanta, or Maalox. Dr. Joel Richter, chairman and professor of gastroenterology at the Cleveland Clinic Foundation, reports that these treatments, plus mucosal protec-

tant medications known as sulcrafates, are safest because they are not sys-
temically absorbed by your body. That means they will never reach your
baby. Plus, many also provide you with an extra supply of calcium—an
added bonus. Talk to your doctor about which of these treatments might
be right for you.

While there are a number of prescription medications designed to
treat heartburn, almost none have been tested in pregnancy. These medications are reserved for use in only the most extreme situations—when
heartburn significantly impairs your ability to eat, for example. The one
heartburn medication you should **never** take while pregnant is nizatidine.
It has been linked to increased risk of miscarriage, birth defects, and still-
births.

PROBLEM #4: LEG CRAMPS, SWELLING, AND VARICOSE VEINS

Beginning sometime in your third trimester, you may start to experience
leg cramps—alone or with swelling in your ankles and feet. This may be
particularly true if you spend significant time standing in one place or
even sitting in one position. One reason, say doctors, is because your
blood volume increases by as much as 40 percent during pregnancy, so
circulation is slowed down—and that can result in swelling. The extra
weight of your growing baby also presses on major blood vessels in your
pelvis, further reducing circulation to your lower half—another reason
legs and feet can swell. While no one is certain if the swelling is related to
the leg cramps, often they can occur together.

Another common pregnancy problem is varicose veins—those
bluish-purple vessels that frequently develop on calves and thighs. Because veins in the legs have to work against gravity to push blood flow
back to the heart, they come equipped with a set of tiny valves that close
between each heartbeat. The valves prevent backward blood flow so circulation to the heart can continue uninterrupted. During pregnancy,
however, a series of physiological changes result in leaky valves. The tiny
shut-off devices don't work as efficiently, so not all of the blood pumps
back to the heart as quickly as it should.

The end result means that more blood pools in your leg veins, which eventually causes them to swell. That swelling causes the formation of the twisted, bulging varicose veins, which can begin appearing anytime from your second trimester on. While the veins may itch or even hurt, they are seldom any cause for alarm and most often disappear in the months following childbirth. You should, however, also be aware that while varicose veins are most visible in the legs, they can also occur in your genital area, particularly in your vulva (see Chapter 2) or, more commonly, your rectum. Varicose veins that appear in this area are known as hemorrhoids— which you'll learn more about in just a few minutes.

Taking Care of Your Pregnant Legs: What to Do

One of the best ways to deal with varicose veins is by wearing support hose or even medical-grade compression stockings. If the veins are not yet visible, wearing the stockings early in pregnancy may prevent them from occurring. If they have already started to appear, the hose are a necessity, since they work by adding the compression that your leg vessels need to keep blood from pooling. If you do wear support hose, be certain to put them on as soon as you wake up—*before* you get out of bed. This will help keep a sudden rush of blood from flooding into your leg veins.

To reduce foot and leg swelling, increase your fluid intake. Doing so will increase circulation and speed the release of salt and other minerals that may be binding water and increasing swelling. What can also help, with not only swelling but with varicose veins as well, is simply getting off your feet. Elevating your tootsies should bring relief in about thirty minutes. If it doesn't, and particularly if any one area of your leg is red, painful to the touch, or feels hot, be certain to your call your doctor. A quick examination will help ensure you don't have any blood clots causing the swelling.

You should also consider taking a few minutes each day to stretch your calf muscles, particularly before bedtime. Doing so can be especially helpful in alleviating nocturnal leg cramps. Also avoid pointing your toes when lying in bed, which can increase leg and foot cramping. If leg cramps are severe, massaging your calf muscles using long circular strokes can help, along with applications of warm, moist heat. Although there have been few studies on leg cramps in pregnancy, some research shows that a calcium deficiency may play a role; so increasing your daily intake of calcium-rich low-fat foods—low-fat ice cream, frozen yogurt, or milk—might also help.

PROBLEM #5: HEMORRHOIDS

When varicose veins occur in or around your rectum, they are known as hemorrhoids. A common pregnancy problem, they often develop as a result of your increased weight, which in turn puts pressure on veins in this area, encouraging inflammation and swelling. They are most common in the third trimester, and constipation—another common pregnancy problem—can increase your risk, particularly if you find yourself straining each time you go to the bathroom. Many women also develop hemorrhoids *after* giving birth, as a result of the intense pushing phase of labor.

During or directly after pregnancy, hemorrhoids can develop either internally or externally. Both types are common. Generally, however, external hemorrhoids cause the most discomfort. Forming near the opening of your rectum, they can be seen as well as felt—and they frequently cause pain, particularly when swelling occurs. External hemorrhoids can also cause extreme itching, which can grow worse right after you have a bowel movement or if you sit for long periods of time. Occasionally external hemorrhoids can also cause bleeding.

Internal hemorrhoids usually can't be seen or felt unless they prolapse, or drop down, from your rectum. When this occurs, many doctors advise applying petroleum jelly and gently trying to tuck them back inside. If this does not work, then it's important that you see your obstetrician. The other hallmark of internal hemorrhoids is that they bleed more often than external ones. This usually occurs in conjunction with a bowel movement, which may be speckled with bright red blood. There may also be blood on the toilet tissue. As alarming as this may be, it's usually nothing to be concerned about. Normally the bleeding stops almost immediately, with only a small loss of blood and no consequences. Still, you should report any such incident to your doctor as soon as possible.

TREATING HEMORRHOIDS: WHAT YOU CAN DO

According to experts from the Mayo Clinic, since constipation is a leading cause of hemorrhoids, adding more fiber to your diet, particularly fresh fruits and vegetables, can help. You can also increase your fluid intake—another important, natural way to reduce constipation and in the process help reduce your risk of hemorrhoids. To reduce swelling and itching, some physicians recommend Tucks witch hazel pads, which you hold on the hemorrhoids for several minutes a few times a day. Other things you can try:

- Keep your rectum as clean as possible. Wash with plain water after each bowel movement.

- Take warm sitz baths, using three to four inches of warm water in a tub or basin to soak your rectum for about ten minutes. You can add oatmeal or baking soda to the water to decrease itching.

- Ice packs and cold compresses can relieve itching and reduce swelling and pain.

- Use only soft, unscented white toilet tissue and wipe gently.

- Avoid straining when going to the bathroom. If a bowel movement is difficult, talk to your doctor about a stool softener or fiber supplement.

- Avoid sitting for long periods of time, particularly on the toilet, since this position allows for extra pressure on the rectum, which can aggravate hemorrhoids or even cause them to form.

High Blood Pressure and Pregnancy: What You Should Know

During a healthy pregnancy, your baby will receive all nutrients and oxygen through your blood, which flows freely from your veins, to the placenta, and, eventually, directly into your baby. To help facilitate this action, your blood pressure usually drops slightly in the second trimester, when your baby is experiencing important developmental gains.

Real Life

WHEN NATURAL ISN'T BETTER FOR TREATING CONSTIPATION

Q: I remember that as a child my grandmother frequently gave us cod liver oil for constipation—and it worked great. Now I'm wondering if I can use this remedy during pregnancy. Since it's all natural, I'm thinking it may be better than any of the medications that are available. Is it safe to use?

A: While it's true cod liver oil is natural, in this instance it's not the best treatment. Research shows it can interfere with the absorption of certain nutrients you need for a healthy pregnancy. If you're looking for a natural treatment, try adding more fluids and particularly more fiber to your diet—or the old standby, prune juice or stewed prunes or apricots, which all work well to relieve constipation. If you just can't get enough fiber in your diet, talk to your doctor about a supplement—Citracel, FiberCon, or Metamucil—but be aware some of these formulas contain high amounts of sugar. Stool softeners such as Colace (ducosate) are often prescribed for constipation occurring after birth and are safe to use during pregnancy as well. In fact, if you check the label of your prenatal vitamins, you may find it's already included. It's often added to formulas to help counter the constipating effects of the vitamin's high iron content.

Normally it comes back to baseline, or just slightly above, during your third trimester, and remains there until you deliver.

In roughly 8 percent of pregnant women, however, things don't go quite as planned. For these women, the third trimester can bring a *dramatic* jump in blood pressure. The result, says Dr. Andrei Rebarber, can be an indication of a potentially life-threatening syndrome known as preeclampsia. If left untreated, preeclampsia can progress to eclampsia, a condition that can lead to brain seizures and be fatal for mother and sometimes baby. The unfortunate part, cautions Dr. Rebarber, is that even if blood pressure *is* controlled, preeclampsia or eclampsia can still occur. "The rise in hypertension is just one of the signs that the syndrome is already under way, so even if you keep blood pressure under control, it's not going to make much difference," he says. Other symptoms of preeclampsia include protein in the urine and acute and rapid swelling, usually in the hands and feet.

Women at greatest risk include those pregnant with multiple babies or those with chronic high blood pressure prior to pregnancy. A bout of preeclampsia in an earlier pregnancy may also increase your risk. The only known treatment for preeclampsia is immediate delivery, usually by cesarean section.

PREVENTING PREECLAMPSIA: HOW VITAMINS CAN HELP

While no one is certain what causes preeclampsia to develop in the first place, some researchers believe genetics may play a role. And studies have shown that there is a gene which appears to control the tendency toward high blood pressure and this gene may also play a role in preeclampsia.

Among the very newest theories, one points to oxidative stress as another culprit—with body-wide damage to blood vessel walls occurring from the same free radical molecules that have been linked to cancer and heart disease. When vessel walls are damaged, it may set the stage for preeclampsia to begin—particularly in women who experienced this syndrome in a previous pregnancy.

The good news: For women at high risk, one of nature's simplest treatments could provide life-saving help. That treatment is antioxidant vitamins: specifically, 400 milligrams of vitamin E and 1,000 milligrams of vitamin C beginning right at the start of your pregnancy. Numerous studies, including research published in the *American Journal of Obstetrics and Gynecology* in 2002, found that not only is this treatment safe, but it appears to be very effective in reducing the risk of preeclampsia, particularly in women who experienced early-onset preeclampsia in a previous pregnancy. Dr. Rebarber reports that his practice is using the vitamin therapy for *any* woman at increased risk, including women pregnant with more than one baby.

Studies conducted by Dr. Ramon D. Hermida at the University of Vigo in Spain found that another simple remedy—100 milligrams of aspirin taken at bedtime—may also help reduce risks. While aspirin is not normally recommended for use in pregnancy, if a woman is at very high risk for preeclampsia, Dr. Hermida says it can help. The key, he says, is to take the aspirin at the right time of the day. In research presented at the May 2002 annual meeting of the American Society of Hypertension, he explained how women who took one aspirin a day upon waking had a 16 percent risk of preeclampsia—about equal to those who took a placebo. But for those who took their aspirin *at night*, before bedtime, the risk of preeclampsia dropped down to just 2 percent. These new findings back up earlier research published in the November 2001 issue of the journal *Obstetrics and Gynecology.* Here researchers from Birmingham Women's Hospital in England found that, overall, women at highest risk for preeclampsia could benefit from low-dose aspirin therapy.

Finally, doctors from the Swedish Medical Center in Seattle found that eating a high-fiber diet during pregnancy may decrease your risk of preeclampsia. In their study, women who consumed 24 or more grams of fiber daily were 51 percent less likely to develop preeclampsia than women who ate just 13 grams of fiber a day.

The important thing to remember is that most women who do develop high blood pressure during pregnancy, and even preeclampsia, *do deliver healthy babies.* The key is to keep in close contact with your doctor and have your blood pressure monitored throughout your pregnancy, particularly if you are at high risk. If you can, monitor your pressure at home, and be certain to call your doctor immediately if it begins to climb.

Whether you are considered at high risk or not, call your doctor immediately if you experience any early signs of preeclampsia: a sudden swelling in the hands, feet, or face, or sudden vision problems. **Do not attempt to treat or prevent preeclampsia on your own, even with seemingly simple treatments like vitamins or aspirin.** If you are at risk, you need the care of a high-risk pregnancy expert or an obstetrician who has experience treating this condition. Your life and your baby's life depend on it.

Blood Sugar and Your Pregnancy

Each year about 200,000 pregnant women experience a problem known as gestational diabetes—a condition that impairs the ability of the hormone insulin to properly move sugar from the blood to the tissues and organs where it is needed to produce energy.

In this condition, women produce *enough* insulin, but its effectiveness is blocked by a series of physiological events linked to pregnancy. This includes the secretion of hormones by the placenta, which actually work to destroy insulin. While in the beginning of pregnancy a woman's natural insulin production overpowers these hormones, somewhere around the twenty-fourth week this can change. As your baby grows, more of these insulin-destroying placental hormones are produced, slowly disabling your body's ability to compensate. "At some point—usually between the twentieth and twenty-fourth week of pregnancy—the hormones overpower the insulin production," says Dr. Loren Wisner-Greene, an endocrinologist at New York University Medical Center. As a result, she says, the body reacts in much the same way it would with diabetes: Levels of blood sugar begin to rise. When this occurs, full-blown gestational diabetes develops.

DIABETES: ARE YOU AT RISK?

According to the American Diabetes Association (ADA), risk factors include obesity, family history of diabetes, previous birth of a large baby or a stillbirth or a child with birth defects, or a condition known as polyhydramnios (too much amniotic fluid). With or without those risk factors, however, the ADA recommends that *all* pregnant women be screened for blood sugar levels at their first prenatal exam. A simple test can tell if you might be at risk, and a second, slightly more complex test can help verify if you do have a problem.

If you are considered at high risk for gestational diabetes, the National Institutes of Health suggests that you get tested twice: first at the very start of your pregnancy and again somewhere between week twenty-four and twenty-eight, even if your first test is negative. If you are at average risk, they suggest testing once, during this later part of your pregnancy. If you are at very low risk, talk to your doctor about whether you need testing.

For many women, symptoms and problems of gestational diabetes can be easily controlled via dietary and lifestyle modifications. You'll need to consume lots of fresh fruits and vegetables (which you should already be doing as part of a healthy pregnancy eating plan), and you will need to avoid certain foods, particularly high-sugar snacks such as cake, cookies, candy, or ice cream. Substituting these foods with wholesome natural snacks such as raisins, carrot sticks, or fruit can be a big help. Complex carbohydrates, such as whole wheat pasta or bread, brown rice, or grains such as oatmeal, can also help control blood sugar.

It's also important not to skip any meals and to eat six small rather than three large meals a day. One of the best things you can do to help not only reduce the risk of gestational diabetes but also control it after it sets in is to watch your weight gain during pregnancy. While you shouldn't be dieting during pregnancy, it's important that you *don't gain* too much weight too quickly and that you control *how much* you gain during each trimester.

What can help in this respect is exercise, and Dr. Wisner-Greene says that increasing your activity level is also a good way to control your blood sugar. Not only will regular exercise—including walking—help keep blood sugar balanced, it can also help you keep your weight under good control.

If, however, sugar levels continue to rise, insulin injections may become necessary. Although oral medications used to treat insulin resistance in Type II diabetes would, at least theoretically, be helpful during pregnancy, Dr. Wisner-Greene reports that, because information on the use of these drugs during pregnancy is limited, they are rarely prescribed for gestational diabetes. This situation, she says, may change in the near future, since one study has already shown that at least one oral medication may work well during pregnancy.

Fortunately, if sugar levels are controlled during pregnancy, gestational diabetes rarely presents any *serious* problems for your baby. It can, however, cause your baby to grow larger than normal—a condition known as "macrosomia," making a cesarean delivery necessary. Your baby

Real Life

IT'S ALL IN THE WRIST

Q: I'm in my second trimester and suddenly my wrist is hurting—so much so that I can no longer work at my computer. I have pain and numbness in my fingers and hand, and it gets worse at night. Is this something I should talk to my OB about, or is it just the usual work strain?

A: What you describe sounds like carpal tunnel syndrome, a nerve compression in the wrist that can affect up to 25 percent of mothers-to-be. The symptoms develop when the hand is overused. As your wrist is continually forced into a bent position—which it can be during computer use—the pathway through which certain key nerves must pass becomes compressed. This causes pressure on the nerves, which accounts for your symptoms. The problem can grow worse in pregnancy due to the same water retention that makes your feet swell. According to Florida orthopedic hand specialist Dr. Deane Carr, using a hand splint—available at most drugstores—can keep your wrist from bending, which will reduce swelling and ultimately nerve inflammation. Ice compresses can also help. A recent medical study found that yoga exercises that strengthen the upper body may relieve carpal tunnel syndrome pain by promoting relaxation of the arm and hand muscles. You may also want to switch from a computer mouse to a touchpad device, like the kind found on laptops, which have been shown to decrease wrist problems. If these measures don't help, talk to your doctor about a local injection of steroids and anesthesia—a drug combination designed to reduce inflammation. The procedure won't harm your baby, but relief is only temporary, so eventually modifying your work routines may be your only answer.

Fortunately, with or without treatment, the problem should completely resolve soon after your baby is born.

---

may also have an increased risk of low blood sugar directly following birth, and an increased risk of jaundice and respiratory distress syndrome (RSD), which can make breathing hard for your newborn. Later in life your child may also have a higher risk of diabetes and obesity.

Real Life

BREATHLESS IN SEATTLE

Q: Is it normal to get out of breath easily during pregnancy? I used to be able to bound up my apartment stairs like a bunny. Now I crawl like a turtle and I'm still out of breath. I am in my fifth month of pregnancy and I am carrying twins.

A: During pregnancy, there are changes in the way your body uses oxygen and carbon dioxide. According to Dr. Gerard Varlotta, a sports medicine physician at New York University Medical Center, the result can be increased respiration—you breathe more quickly and less deeply. Both can contribute to feelings of breathlessness. Making matters just a little worse, he says, is pressure on your diaphragm from your expanding uterus. Not surprisingly, this situation occurs more frequently in a multiple pregnancy.

Although it can be frustrating, this problem is not generally dangerous and often improves during the last few weeks of pregnancy, when your baby drops farther into your pelvis, relieving pressure on your diaphragm. In the meantime, concentrate on posture—sitting and standing as straight as you can. Lying on your left side with your legs propped on a pillow can help as well. Most important, says Dr. Varlotta, don't push yourself; if you must move slower, do so, and don't compete with what you were able to accomplish before getting pregnant.

There is, however, one additional word of warning: Sometimes anemia—caused by a reduced level of red blood cells—can result in fatigue and that feeling of being out of breath, particularly upon exertion. During pregnancy, your blood volume increases by almost 50 percent—but most of that increase is due to *blood plasma,* and not *red blood cells.* In about 20 percent of women, the first half of pregnancy results in a low red blood count and some of the symptoms you describe. If, however, you are eating nutritiously and taking a prenatal vitamin with extra iron, anemia is not likely to be a problem. To be certain you are okay, ask your doctor about a complete blood count (CBC)—a test that will show your level of red and white cells. If you are anemic, eating more red meat and taking extra vitamin B_{12} and iron can help.

> ## Real Life

SQUINTING TO SEE THE LIGHT

Q: I wear contact lenses for distance viewing and have had the same prescription for years. But since becoming pregnant, suddenly my vision has declined—I don't see as clearly, and I am also having trouble reading, which I never had before. I had my eyes checked right before I got pregnant and everything was fine. Is it possible something really serious has gone wrong now?

A: While it's always possible that your vision problems could be a symptom of something else—including an early sign of pregnancy-related high blood pressure—chances are they stem from fluid retention. This puts pressure on your eyeball, causing temporary vision changes during pregnancy. You can, however, talk to your doctor about eye relief products such as Visine. **Note:** If your vision changes dramatically or suddenly, call your doctor right away.

Generally, your blood sugar levels will return to normal shortly after birth. However, a recent study *has* shown that approximately half of the women who develop gestational diabetes go on to develop Type II insulin-resistant diabetes within fifteen years of giving birth. According to Dr. Wisner-Greene, checking blood sugar six weeks after giving birth can predict whether you are at future risk. If you are diagnosed with gestational diabetes, it's a good idea to have your blood sugar checked at your six-week postpartum visit, as well as during your annual physical.

Vaginal Bleeding: What You Need to Know

Among the most common and frightening of pregnancy problems is vaginal bleeding, particularly when it occurs early in pregnancy. As scary as it can be, however, most of the time there is no cause for alarm. Many women experience some level of vaginal spotting or bleeding in the first trimester without any reason or any risk of complication.

That said, according to the American College of Obstetricians and

Real Life

SINKING YOUR TEETH IN

Q: I am in my second trimester and I've begun developing these tiny little bumps on my gums, which are also very red and bleed almost every time I brush my teeth. I called my dentist and he said there is nothing to worry about—it's normal in pregnancy. But without an exam, I'm concerned that he might be missing something more serious. I've never heard of "gum bumps" as a part of pregnancy—and wonder if it's generally safe to get dental work done during this time.

A: The problem here could be what dentists call pyogenic granulomas, more commonly known as *pregnancy tumors*. But don't let the phrase scare you. These are generally harmless, noncancerous growths that spontaneously occur during pregnancy and disappear shortly after giving birth.

Of greater concern is your red and bleeding gums, which could be the result of pregnancy gingivitis—a gum inflammation that can appear as early as the second month of pregnancy and often peaks in the eighth month. According to Dr. Kim Loos, dental instructor at the Pacific School of Dentistry in San Jose, California, the problem is usually the result of an increase in estrogen and progesterone—and it should definitely not be ignored.

Studies show that, when left untreated, the bacteria associated with gum disease can travel through your bloodstream to your uterus, increasing the risk of infection, which in turn increases your risk of preterm labor. Getting treatment, however, can turn your risks around. In research published in August 2002 in the *Journal of Periodontology*, doctors report that women who do receive treatment for gum disease during pregnancy often reduce their risk of having a low-birthweight or preterm baby by a significant margin. And while most doctors advise pregnant women to hold off on any dental work that isn't considered an emergency, a simple checkup and routine cleaning, particularly during mid-pregnancy, can help ensure teeth and gums remain healthy.

Gynecologists, there are a number of conditions in which bleeding *may* represent a problem, including an increased risk of miscarriage. This is more likely the case if your bleeding is accompanied by cramping. Although sometimes pregnancy loss is nature's way of dealing with an unhealthy conception, just as often the symptoms serve as a simple warning that some type of auxiliary treatment may be necessary to sustain your pregnancy. The only way to know for certain is to call your doctor as soon as possible whenever cramping and/or bleeding occur.

In most instances, you will be asked to go to your doctor's office for a medical evaluation, which usually includes a pelvic exam, a blood test for hCG (human chorionic gonadotropin), and sometimes a sonogram. These tests are particularly important since occasionally bleeding and cramping can also result from an ectopic pregnancy—a condition in which a fertilized embryo is stuck within the fallopian tube and cannot reach your uterus. Affecting about one in every sixty pregnancies, this is considered a life-threatening medical emergency and requires that your pregnancy be terminated in order to ensure your safety. Fortunately, most of the time, an ectopic pregnancy is *not* the cause of your vaginal bleeding. In most women, bleeding and cramping will stop on their own and no further treatment will be needed. If a miscarriage is a possibility, your doctor may prescribe something as simple as bed rest or possibly medications designed to strengthen your uterus and stop contractions.

If you cannot reach your doctor after cramping and bleeding have begun, go directly to the nearest hospital emergency room and tell them you are pregnant.

BLEEDING IN LATE PREGNANCY: WHAT YOU SHOULD KNOW

Bleeding that occurs in the second half of pregnancy represents a completely different set of circumstances and usually requires different kinds of treatment. One common cause of minor bleeding in your second or third trimester can be an inflamed cervix, in which case treatment is not usually required.

But when *heavy* vaginal bleeding occurs, it can be more serious, often involving a problem with the placenta. Most commonly, this includes placental abruption, in which your baby's birth sac separates from your uterus, and placenta previa, when the birth sac drops low in the uterus and covers the cervix. According to studies, placental abruption occurs in about 1 percent of women, usually taking place sometime during the last twelve weeks of the pregnancy. When the degree of separation is slight, nothing more than bed rest may be required. If, however, the separation is significant, your baby could experience critical oxygen deprivation—which often facilitates the need for an immediate cesarean delivery.

Although sometimes bleeding from placental abruption can be extremely heavy—marking a true hospital emergency—just as often it can be very slight. Interestingly, the level at which you bleed does not predict the extent of the separation—another reason why even small amounts of vaginal bleeding late in your pregnancy should be reported to your doctor as soon as possible.

When placenta previa occurs, your embryo attaches to your uterine wall in a lower than normal location. In many instances your doctor can spot this early on in your pregnancy. As your baby grows and moves, the misplaced placental sac becomes dislodged, a problem that can cause significant, painless bleeding some time after the twentieth week of pregnancy. During your third trimester you are likely to experience three such bleeding episodes, frequently with significant blood loss.

For many women, bleeding very late in pregnancy can be a sign that labor is beginning! As the tiny mucous plug that has been sealing off the opening of your uterus becomes dislodged, a small amount of blood—called the bloody show—may occur. If you begin to see light vaginal bleeding close to your due date, it is likely a sign that labor *is* about to start. If it happens earlier, however, you may be experiencing premature labor—and you should call your doctor immediately.

Coping with Pregnancy Emergencies: What to Do

Besides bleeding, there are a number of other key symptoms you should be aware of—problems that might require some quick medical attention. To help you pinpoint when it's really essential to reach your doctor right away, check out this symptom list. Compiled with the help of experts from the Minnesota Women's Health Consortium, Planned Parenthood, and the University of California at Irvine Medical Group, it can help you spot trouble, get treatment, and prevent any major problems from occurring. Also remember that while not all symptoms are indicative of a serious concern, they do represent the potential for problems, so they should never be ignored.

When to Call Your Doctor Immediately

✓ Leaking fluid from your vagina—blood or a clear fluid

✓ Unusual or severe abdominal or back pain

✓ Sudden swelling in hands, feet, or face

✓ Contraction-like pains

✓ Sudden weight gain of two pounds or more in one day

✓ Blurry or impaired vision that occurs suddenly

When to Call Your Doctor as Soon as Possible

✓ Excessive vomiting or diarrhea

✓ Persistent chills

✓ Fever of 101 degrees or higher

✓ Increased thirst with decreased urination

✓ Severe or unusual headaches

✓ Appearance of genital sores or warts

✓ Fainting spells

When to Head for the Hospital Immediately

✓ Significant vaginal bleeding or hemorrhage

✓ Inability to tolerate any food or liquid for more than twenty-four hours

✓ Severe abdominal pain

✓ Sudden loss of vision, numbness, or pain down one side of your body

✓ Abdominal pain that recurs every five to ten minutes

Your Intimate Pregnancy

A V Zone and Breast Care Guide

Among the many changes that will occur in your body, pregnancy can bring about some significant differences in your intimate anatomy. From a new and more abundant vaginal discharge, to increased urination and sometimes problems controlling the flow, to changes in the size, shape, and feel of your breasts, there's no question that the most private parts of your body are going to begin looking, feeling, and acting significantly different. At times, the changes can seem so profound, you may even begin to feel as if you are living in someone else's body!

Complicating matters a bit further, you may find that at least some of the ways in which you normally care for your intimate anatomy—particularly in regard to hygiene practices—suddenly don't work anymore. You may even find yourself concerned with products and ingredients you've used for years, wondering if they are safe while baby is in tow. Even simple practices you took for granted just yesterday—like bikini waxing or using a vaginal deodorant—may suddenly seem a cause for concern.

The good news is that few if any of the V zone problems you will experience during pregnancy are any real cause for alarm. Many are a typical part of having a baby, and even those that are not don't usually represent any serious threats. Yet that doesn't mean they won't cause you at least some measure of discomfort—and, sometimes, a fair amount of anxiety as well.

The important thing to remember is that with a little bit of knowledge and some good advice, you can not only understand your pregnant V zone better, you can cope with any problems that come your way.

Understanding Your Intimate Anatomy: What You Need to Know

Among the first intimate changes you may notice during pregnancy is how different your vulva and vagina look and feel. One of the most noticeable of these changes is an increase in the production of vaginal discharge. Medically known as leukorrhea, it is essentially the same clear, slippery fluid that your body normally produces to help keep your vagina clean and well lubricated. However, during pregnancy a combination of cervical changes, including an increased blood supply to your vagina, *and* increased stimulation from pressure on your cervix, can double or even triple your amount of vaginal discharge. If you are pregnant with twins, triplets, or quadruplets, your discharge can increase so much that you might feel a distinct sense of wetness through most of your pregnancy.

During your first and second trimesters, you can expect your discharge to be the same clear or white fluid you had before pregnancy, with no strong or noticeable odors. On your panties or panty liner, however, it may take on a slight yellow tinge after it dries. This is perfectly normal. Occasionally it may also take on a slight brownish tint, usually indicative of "old blood" that may have come from your uterus. While it's most often nothing to worry about, if you do see a brownish discharge, check with your doctor, just to be certain.

If at any time during your pregnancy your discharge takes on a foul or "fishy" odor, or if it dramatically changes color, to green, yellow, or gray, or if it becomes frothy and white in appearance, it's important to see your doctor, since these could be signs of a V zone infection that requires medical care. (See Chapter 11 for additional information on vaginal infections during pregnancy.)

As your pregnancy progresses into the third trimester and you get closer to your due date, discharge will become even more abundant and, often, thicker. As early as two weeks before labor begins, you may suddenly notice *a lot* more mucus. If so, it's probably the breakdown of your mucous plug, a thick seal that forms over your cervix and blocks anything from entering your uterus during pregnancy. When this occurs you may even see a little blood—something doctors call the "bloody show" or show—a sign that labor will be starting soon.

IMPORTANT: Call your doctor as soon as you see any amount of blood in your discharge, regardless of what point you are in your pregnancy. While it's most likely nothing to worry about, your doctor may want to see you, just to check that no treatment is needed to ensure the health of your baby.

Yeast Infections and Your Pregnancy

It itches; it burns; and it causes a cheesy white discharge that can leave you feeling wet and uncomfortable all the time. The problem is a yeast infection, and it is among the most common V zone problems to occur during pregnancy. Why?

Normally, vaginal health is kept in check by a highly precise feminine ecosystem—a network of physiological activity that helps maintain balance among the many microorganisms present in your tissues, including candidiasis, the fungus that causes a yeast infection. However, the flurry of hormonal activity that occurs during pregnancy can change that balance, allowing candidiasis to begin multiplying rapidly. Further, some believe that because pregnancy has an impact on the immune system, slightly compromising your body's natural biochemical balance, organisms like yeast may grow out of control more quickly and easily. If you also happen to be suffering from external hemorrhoids—which frequently harbor yeast—a vaginal infection can set in even sooner or be more difficult to treat.

Although generally yeast infections pose no major threat to your

Real Life

AMNIOCENTESIS AND VAGINAL DISCHARGE

Q: I had an amniocentesis, and for several days afterward I had an extremely heavy vaginal discharge—more so than usual. I didn't tell my doctor, but now I'm thinking maybe I should have. Could this have been a sign that something went wrong?

A: Amniocentesis is a test in which your doctor inserts an ultra-thin needle through your navel to extract a sample of the amniotic fluid that surrounds your baby in the womb. Since the fluid contains cells from your baby, it is used to check for developmental abnormalities—and it is generally a safe test that does not cause any problems. Because, however, it does involve a puncture into the amniotic fluid sac, sometimes a heavy or unusually wet discharge following the test signals a leak has occurred. According to Dr. Steve Goldstein, professor of obstetrics and gynecology at New York University Medical Center, most often the problem will repair itself. However, it's still important that you call your doctor immediately if you experience wetness following an amniocentesis. Most likely, she or he will suggest nothing more than bed rest for a day or two, to give your uterus time to heal. However, should the extra discharge continue, or if it is initially very heavy, you should be checked by your doctor, to ensure an infection has not developed.

baby, if the fungus is out of control at the time you deliver, there is a small chance your baby may contract a disease known as thrush. This is an oral yeast infection categorized by small white patches on the inside of the mouth. Even if this should occur, however, treatment is fast, safe, and easy.

TREATING YOUR YEAST INFECTION: WHAT TO DO

While a yeast infection itself remains the same in pregnant and nonpregnant women, what changes is how it's treated. That's because at least some of the medications may cause problems for developing babies. At least one commonly prescribed yeast infection treatment—the oral medication Diflucan (fluconazole)—should not be used during pregnancy at all. According to Dr. William Ledger, chief of obstetrics and gynecology at New York Weill Cornell Medical Center in New York City, treatments that are considered safer include over-the-counter products such as Monistat and Gyne-Lotrimin, as well as prescription drugs Terazol and Nystatin (mycostatin) in vaginal tablet form.

But before you head for the drugstore, remember that your baby's stage of development is key to choosing a treatment option. Thus, even seemingly safe topical drugs are frequently not recommended for use during the first trimester—a critical growth stage for your baby. In fact, many doctors believe that only two yeast infection treatments are safe to use in early pregnancy: gentian violet and mycostatin. Unfortunately, both have lower-than-normal success rates. If your symptoms do not clear with these medications, many doctors suggest you wait until later in your pregnancy before seeking more aggressive treatment.

If, however, a yeast infection develops in your second or third trimester, you will have more treatment options. Still, nearly all doctors agree that the less time you spend on medication, the better it is for your baby. Therefore, most recommend the three-day treatment regimen. While one-day treatments are available, if you have any sensitivity to these drugs, the concentrated amount of medication in these pills may be more likely to increase your risk of a negative reaction.

YEAST INFECTION RED ALERTS

· Never self-treat a yeast infection during pregnancy, even if you have had a similar infection in the past. Sometimes yeast infections can be confused with a normal increase in vaginal secretions or potentially more serious vaginal infections. The bottom line: Always consult with your doctor before deciding on any treatment.

· Sometimes, continuing bouts of yeast infections in pregnancy signal the onset of gestational diabetes, a serious pregnancy complication. For this reason, make certain your doctor knows about any yeast infections you do develop and discuss the need for blood sugar testing. (See Chapter 1.)

Mother *Nature* Knows Best

ALL-NATURAL YEAST INFECTION TREATMENTS

For all-natural relief from yeast infection symptoms, you can safely try:

- Witch hazel compresses or ice packs to calm inflamed vaginal tissue.

- Aveeno Colloidal Oatmeal or 2 cups of cornstarch plus ½ cup of baking soda in a tub of warm water; soak for ten minutes.

- Local applications of nonflavored, unsweetened yogurt; eating more yogurt.

- Cotton underwear. And spend at least several hours a day without panties, allowing maximum air circulation to your vagina.

- Homeopathic Vagisil Yeast Itch Control Suppositories—but get your doctor's okay first.

More Vaginal Infections and Pregnancy: What You Must Know

While yeast infections remain among the most common V zone problems to develop during pregnancy, others can rear their ugly heads during this time as well, often when you least expect it. Among those affecting a significant number of women is bacterial vaginosis (BV), an umbrella term that is frequently used to cover a number of infections that can invade the vagina. Although BV can sometimes produce symptoms—including burning, itching, discharge, or even pain—just as often it can be silent. Many women don't even know they have BV until it's revealed during their prenatal exam.

In the early 1990s, studies strongly suggested that any BV infection in pregnancy, even those that caused no symptoms, could increase the risk of premature birth. As a result, there was an urgency to treat

Real Life

V ZONE VARICOSE VEINS

Q: I am pregnant with my fourth child, and I notice a swelling in my vaginal lips that comes and goes. When it swells, the pain is horrific— it's a heavy, aching kind of pain. I have checked for lumps or bumps and don't feel anything—but it hurts the worst when I am walking or standing. Whenever I'm due for a doctor's visit, it seems to go away. What could be causing this?

A: Whether your problem is occurring at the time you see your doctor or not, you should always discuss during your prenatal exam any troubling symptoms you are experiencing. That said, your symptoms could be an indication of vulvar varicosite—or what you may normally know of as varicose veins. Although they usually occur in the legs—appearing as bulging blue veins—they can also develop in your vulva, with little or no discoloration seen on the outside. Varicose veins that develop in and around your rectum are known as hemorrhoids. (See Chapter 1.)

Vulvar varicosites are generally caused by an increase in circulation to the entire pelvic area. This increases the likelihood that blood will pool in the tiny vessels inside your vulva, causing the swelling and fullness you describe. When you walk or stand, pressure on the veins increases, and so does the discomfort. Unlike the veins in your legs, however, which generally appear blue and bulging, the veins in your V zone may appear normal to the eye, so you *feel* the pressure but may not necessarily *see* the discoloration.

Among the best treatments: a cool compress, which can reduce swelling and pain. Staying off your feet can help as well, although total relief probably won't come until baby is born. That's when the veins usually revert back to normal.

any pregnant woman found to harbor a BV infection, even if she had no symptoms.

Today, however, this is no longer the case. Newer and more reliable research has shown that treating asymptomatic BV infections does not reduce the risk of preterm labor or early delivery. This remains the case for both women at high risk for these problems and those at low risk or no risk.

The same is true for Trichomonas, another vaginal infection previously linked to preterm labor. In fact, one study revealed that women who were treated for Trichomonas during pregnancy actually ended up at *greater* risk for premature birth.

Today most doctors do not offer pregnant women treatment for these infections, even if a problem is found during a pelvic exam. If, however, you are experiencing symptoms that are making your pregnancy uncomfortable, don't hesitate to talk to your doctor about which medications may help you.

THE V ZONE TEST YOU MUST NOT SKIP

While it may be considered safe to let BV or even trichomonas go untreated during pregnancy, the one vaginal infection you should never ignore is GBS—short for Group B Streptococcus. A common bacteria, it can be found in the vagina or the lower intestines of up to 35 percent of women. While some experience bladder or uterine infections related to Strep B, many women experience no symptoms at all—and most don't even know they are harboring the bacteria. And if you aren't pregnant, it doesn't really matter.

Once you conceive, however, the risk profile changes dramatically, because GBS can be *deadly* to your baby. Exposure during the birthing process (when babies can either inhale or swallow the bacteria) can lead to a life-threatening blood infection (sepsis) or meningitis, an infection of the fluid and lining surrounding the brain.

According to the March of Dimes, if you carry the GBS bacteria in your vagina or rectum at the time of your delivery, your baby has a 1 in 100 chance of becoming infected. While many babies who *are* infected have no long-lasting damage, the potential for serious consequences is always present. Studies show that up to 5 percent of all newborns infected with GBS die, while up to 30 percent suffer serious neurological damage.

In the past, only those women at high risk for GBS were tested prior to delivery: those who went into labor before thirty-seven weeks, ruptured their membrane eighteen hours or more before labor began, or had a temperature of 100.4 degrees or more during labor. Women who previously gave birth to a baby with GBS, or those who had a GBS-related urinary tract infection during pregnancy, were also considered at risk and usually offered the test, which consists of a simple swabbing of the vagina and rectum.

Now, however, some experts are calling for a change. In October 2002 the National Centers for Disease Control issued an advisory suggesting that *all* pregnant women be routinely tested for GBS between the thirty-fifth and thirty-seventh week of pregnancy—a policy that doctors are being urged to adopt. Right now, however, it may be up to you to ask for the test or even insist on it late in your third trimester. If you do test positive, you have the option of being treated with intravenous antibiotics during labor, which studies show can dramatically decrease your baby's risk of infection.

The V Zone Massage:
How to Make Childbirth Easier

During childbirth, the area between your vagina and your rectum, called the perineum, will stretch to remarkable proportions. Although this tissue is highly elastic, it still can tear during childbirth. To keep that from happening, doctors sometimes perform a procedure known as a episiotomy—a cutting of the perineum—which some say heals easier than a tear.

However, at least some research shows that massaging the perineum during pregnancy, particularly in the last six weeks, can help condition and stretch tissues, allowing for easier childbirth, less risk of tearing, and reduced need for an episiotomy. In studies published in 1999 in the journal *Obstetrics and Gynecology*, doctors noted that just five to ten minutes of perineal massage daily can help make childbirth far easier, particularly in women experiencing a first-time vaginal birth. A study of nearly 400 pregnant women published in the *Journal of Obstetrics, Gynecology and Neonatal Nursing* in 2000 found that perineal massage reduces the overall incidence of V zone lacerations during childbirth and makes labor and delivery easier.

Although there are various ways to do a perineal massage and a number of different techniques, many doctors, including the researchers who conducted these studies, recommend the following steps:

1. Empty your bladder and wash your hands.

2. Prop up your body on pillows so that your hands can comfortably reach the inside of your vagina.

3. Apply a mild lubricant, such as sweet almond oil or wheatgerm oil, to your hands. Insert one or two fingers up to 3 centimeters (or 1 inch) inside your vagina and apply pressure, pressing downward toward your rectum, creating a stretching sensation.

4. As you maintain pressure, begin massaging using U-shape movements, then hold the stretch for thirty to sixty seconds and release.

5. Massage with more oil, stretch again, hold and release. Repeat for five to ten minutes.

If your nails are very long, take care not to scratch your vulva or vagina during the massage. Wearing latex medical grade gloves can help.

While massaging, experts suggest trying to stretch your vagina until you feel a tingling sensation inside your muscles. This is similar to what you may feel when your baby's head begins to descend during delivery. While experiencing the "burn," tighten your pelvic muscles—the same ones you use to stop urinating midstream. You will notice that the pain intensifies. Then relax those same muscles until the pain stops, and try to remember how your body feels when you do this.

The ability to relax your pelvic muscles during childbirth will prove very helpful in avoiding tissue damage and perineal tears. Knowing how it feels when these muscles are relaxed can help you to duplicate the moves during childbirth.

To help increase relaxation prior to massage, try soaking in a warm tub for about ten minutes. Also note that, while your muscles might feel tight when you start the massage, generally it should not cause you any significant pain. If a perineal massage is significantly painful, mention it to your doctor long before your due date.

Bladder Control and Pregnancy: What You Need to Know

Among the most common intimate care problems associated with pregnancy has to do with incontinence—a leaking of urine that can develop, particularly during the latter half of pregnancy. Why does this occur?

Anatomically speaking, your uterus lies just above your bladder, which is where urine collects just prior to urination. As your baby grows and your uterus increases in size, it presses on your bladder, making it unable to hold as much urine as it did before. Additionally, increased blood flow to the entire pelvic region can make your bladder "feel" full even when it isn't. If that weren't enough, the extra blood volume that occurs during pregnancy means you actually produce more urine at this time.

All things considered, it's not hard to see why you may feel the urge to urinate more often than you ever did before. But more importantly, at least from a hygiene standard, is that you may also be plagued with something called stress incontinence—urine "leaks" that are the result of the extra stress that occurs whenever you cough, laugh, or sneeze. Usually this happens more frequently in the first trimester, when the position of your womb is putting direct pressure on your bladder, and again in your third trimester, when you baby's position changes and pressure increases once again.

The best way to deal with bladder control problems is, of course, to prevent them as much as you can. One of the best ways you can do that is via pelvic exercises known as Kegels, movements that are designed to strengthen the muscles that hold up your bladder. Beginning Kegel exercises anytime during your pregnancy can make a significant difference. You'll find information on how to do a Kegel, as well as some additional pelvic exercises, in Chapter 5.

In addition, you may find that urinating more frequently can help. If you don't let your bladder get too full, you'll be less likely to experience "accidents" or leaks. What you must never do is restrict fluid intake to control incontinence. It is essential that you drink at least eight glasses of water a day, and more if your pregnancy stretches over a long, hot summer. What you *can* do is avoid fluids one to two hours before bedtime. This can cut down on nighttime bathroom trips and possibly help you sleep better.

If, however, you find that urine leaks or drips are still a problem, consider using urinary incontinence pads to catch dribbles and drips. While you may think that products like Poise and Depend are only for older folks, they can be a real blessing during pregnancy. Designed to hold more liquid than a sanitary pad, the products also help keep wetness away from your body, which may, in turn, help you avoid local vulvar irritation. Although most of these pads contain some form of odor control, dousing them with cornstarch will help further reduce odors and keep wetness away from your body.

In the later stages of your pregnancy—particularly the last four weeks of your third trimester—be certain you don't confuse incontinence with your water breaking, an event that signals the start of labor. In this instance, it is not urine that is flowing, but the fluid that filled the amniotic sac in which your baby developed and grew. While many women expect that their water breaking will cause an unmistakable gush of fluid, this is not always the case. Sometimes it could be a slow trickle and may seem as if you are only leaking urine. There is, however, a way to tell the difference.

When It's Your Water Breaking: You're more likely to feel the sudden wetness when you stand up, especially after sitting or lying down for a while. This will occur even if you move slowly and carefully. In addition, the fluid is usually colorless and odorless, and may contain tiny specks of mucus or even blood.

When It's Urine Leaking: You will feel the wetness most when you cough, laugh, sneeze, or anytime you move, even when you are lying down. Additionally, urine has a yellow tinge and usually has some odor, most often an ammonia-like smell.

Real Life

TIPPED UTERUS AND URINATION

Q: I always heard that women experience an increased urge to urinate when they are pregnant, but I have just the opposite. I am in my first trimester and have a very hard time urinating, even when I feel the urge. I never had this before—and I'm wondering if it means something is wrong, since I was also diagnosed with a tipped uterus.

A: Experts say that if your uterus is reverted, or "tipped" backward, instead of putting pressure on your bladder, it compresses the urethra, a tiny tube that carries urine from your bladder out of your body. The compression works to "seal off" or reduce the function of the urethra, making it harder to urinate.

The good news is that after the first trimester, the position of your uterus changes and the pressure on your urethra may be reduced, making urination easier. If it doesn't, your doctor can insert a device known as a pessary—a rubber doughnut that is used to elevate the uterus and relieve the pressure on the urethra.

Another consideration: Sometimes fibroid tumors can grow quite large during pregnancy. Depending on where they are located, they might cause a blockage that makes it more difficult to urinate. If problems urinating become severe, or if they don't improve by your second trimester, you should talk to your doctor. Normally, you should urinate at least three to six times (or more) in a twenty-four-hour period.

Remember, it's important to call your doctor anytime you experience a significant loss of fluid, particularly late in your pregnancy. Once your water breaks, you and your baby are much more vulnerable to infection, and you'll need your doctor's care and advice.

WHEN BLADDER CONTROL PROBLEMS MEAN
SOMETHING MORE

Among the most common medical problems occurring during pregnancy is a urinary tract infection (UTI). By some accounts, up to 7 percent of all pregnant women will experience one or more UTIs and will need a round of antibiotics for treatment. Often, however, UTIs can be overlooked at their earliest, most easily treated stages. The reason: One of the most prominent symptoms—a frequent urge to urinate—is confused with the normal urge for frequent urination that occurs during pregnancy. There is, however, an easy way to tell the difference: If your urge to urinate is also accompanied by discomfort, including burning or pain—particularly cramping just above your bikini line during or right after urination—then a UTI should be suspected. Additionally, a UTI may also cause you to have tinges of blood or actual blood in your urine, a slight fever, and an all-over achy feeling. Pressure from pregnancy alone won't do that.

Most often your obstetrician will test you for a urinary infection on your first prenatal visit. And if you *are* infection free at that time, it's doubtful that you will have any problems later in your pregnancy. What can increase that risk, however, is a history of chronic UTIs—in which case you should be retested at least once every trimester. If it turns out you do have an infection, it is imperative that you take whatever antibiotic your doctor prescribes.

While most physicians like to avoid prescribing drugs in pregnancy, research presented at the first Centers for Disease Control and Prevention Conference on Birth Defects in October 2002 is changing many a medical mind. Here, researchers from the University of South Carolina presented a study on some 80,000 women, revealing that when UTIs remain untreated during pregnancy, the baby's risk of mental retardation increased by a whopping 40 percent. According to lead researcher Dr. Suzanne McDermott, the good news is that researchers found *no links to retardation* when medication was taken to abate the infection.

That said, if you do develop a UTI during pregnancy, **never** take any medications from a previous infection—or have a prescription refilled— without checking with your doctor first. While some of the drugs normally used to treat UTIs are safe during pregnancy, many are not. Only your doctor can advise you on the best medication for you. Once a drug is prescribed, don't be afraid to take it.

Your Pregnant Breasts: What You Can Expect

If you've ever wondered how you might look and feel with substantially larger breasts, pregnancy is the time to try on your new look! In fact, most women add between one and two pounds of weight to *each* breast during pregnancy—and some are quite surprised that the "growth spurt" occurs as quickly as it does, with most of the change occurring in the first trimester.

One reason for that growth spurt is that from almost the moment you conceive, your breasts begin setting the stage for milk production. As estrogen and progesterone levels soar, they combine with the hormone human placental lactogen (HPL), as well as thyroid hormone, to stimulate the growth of a tiny network of vessels called milk ducts. As the duct system grows, so do your breasts. Eventually they will develop enough to carry milk made deep inside your breasts out to your nipples, where it can be expressed during feeding.

But size isn't the only change caused by the developing ducts. As they grow, they can compress nerve endings located deep inside each breast. This increases breast sensitivity, sometimes causing a burning or tingling sensation, leaving you feeling tender and painful to the touch. Sometimes the area around your nipples may even become significantly inflamed.

All these problems can be made worse by intimate contact—which may become extremely difficult during your first trimester. Fortunately, however, the inflammation doesn't last long. By the start of the second trimester, your breasts should begin feeling more normal and sometimes even more sensuous to the touch. Indeed, the same compressed nerve endings that caused pain in your first trimester may bring about very *pleasurable* sensations in your second trimester.

As your pregnancy progresses, you can also expect your nipples to get larger and firmer, as well as darker in color. This includes the areola, the patch of darkened skin that surrounds your nipple. Although sun expo-

An Expert's Opinion on

COPING WITH BREAST PAIN

For many women, reducing first-trimester breast pain can be as simple as wearing a soft but supportive bra, reports nurse/midwife Barbara Good, from Takoma Women's Health Center in Maryland. In fact, if you normally wear thin, flimsy lingerie, now is the time to invest in not only a new, larger bra, but one that is a bit more substantial in terms of construction. This can help support breast ligaments during the day and at night, and may help ease pain.

To make sure your bra is not *contributing* to your breast pain, check the inside and make certain there are no seams or decorations pushing against your skin. If there is an underwire, make certain it's well padded so it does not cause any friction. According to Good, applying a warm hot-water bottle or warm compress can help breast pain—as long as you don't put it on your stomach or you don't keep it on your breast too long. You can also try reducing salt intake, since, much like during your premenstrual time, the hormones of early pregnancy can cause water retention and bloating, which increases breast tenderness and sensitivity. Cutting down on salty foods will help reduce water retention, which may also help ease some of your breast pain.

sure can promote the darkening, even if your chest never sees the light of day, you can still expect a color change that, for the most part, will be permanent.

BREAST LUMPS, BUMPS, AND LEAKS: WHAT TO DO

Along with changes in breast size, shape, and color come changes in the texture of your breast skin. Most noticeable will probably be the tiny bumps that begin appearing around your nipples, usually beginning in the second trimester. These "bumps" are actually an enlargement of the Montgomery glands, which also grow in response to pregnancy. As they do, they secrete a fluid that has both lubricating

Real Life

CLEAN BREASTS AND PREGNANCY

Q: Is it true that you are not supposed to use soap on your breasts during pregnancy? A friend told me soap was the worst thing I could use to bathe during pregnancy, particularly my breasts. Is this true—and if so, why?

A: Breast hygiene is important. Unfortunately, soap and hot water in particular are anything but gentle or kind to breast skin. The reason: Both can wash away the clear fluid that the nipples naturally secrete to help keep them soft and supple. Soaps, particularly those with no buffers or moisturizers, can easily strip away this natural protection, leaving your breasts susceptible to dryness, itching, and flaking. Your skin may even crack and become inflamed. Conversely, washing your breasts with warm water only—no soap, no cleansers—and lightly towel drying can preserve the natural lubrication that will keep skin softer and less painful during pregnancy and after delivery. This is particularly important if you plan on breast-feeding, since often nipples can become sore and cracked during the first few days. Anything you can do beforehand to condition them can pay off once breast-feeding begins.

and antibacterial properties, and can help keep your nipples soft and supple for breast-feeding.

Additionally, as your breasts prepare to produce milk, sometime in your third trimester, you may also notice your nipples releasing a clear yellowish liquid known as *colostrum*. While for some women this leakage is hardly noticeable and some don't get any at all, for others it can be quite heavy, most often increasing after a warm shower or when breasts are stimulated during intimate activity.

Although it can be frightening when it first occurs, it's important to remember that it's a normal part of pregnancy and no cause for alarm. If you do experience heavy leakage during the day, you may want to invest in some soft, absorbent breast pads. Much like sanitary napkins, they are disposable and tuck discreetly inside your bra.

Occasionally, in addition to the clear yellow breast discharge of colostrum, some women also express a slightly bloody liquid from their nipples. Although it may seem dangerous, it too can be a normal consequence of your growing breasts and no cause for alarm. While you should bring any bloody breast discharge to the attention of your doctor, don't be surprised if she or he does little in the way of testing or treatment. According to breast surgeon Dr. Carol E. H. Scott-Conner from the University of Iowa School of Medicine, because cells in the breast normally change and grow during pregnancy, the results of any tests—such as a biopsy for abnormal breast cells—can be misleading. She says that most of the time, observation and reassurance are appropriate. You won't need further testing she says, unless the problem persists two or more months *after* delivery.

THE RED, WHITE, AND BLUE: STRETCH MARKS AND YOUR BREASTS

Depending on how quickly your breasts increase in size, and the extent of that increase, you may be plagued with reddish blue lines known as stretch marks. While normally they develop on the stomach (and you'll learn more about that in Chapter 3), they can also occur to a slightly lesser extent on the breasts. What may help: wearing a good support bra, not only during the day but also while you sleep. In fact, many experts believe that the more support a breast has, the less likely it is for skin layers to pull and separate, one factor involved in the formation of stretch marks. Additionally, wearing a soft sleep bra at night can help prevent gravity from pulling on breast tissue, thereby reducing skin stretching even more.

Another plus: Wearing a good, sturdy, supportive bra *during the daytime* can pay off after baby is born by reducing the amount of natural sagging that occurs after pregnancy. Wearing a supportive bra during exercise is also important, since it not only can minimize breast pain, but also keep supporting ligaments from being stressed. (See Chapter 4 for more information on pregnancy undergarments.)

And while there is no *scientific* proof that keeping skin on the breast moist will help, anecdotally doctors report that women who do keep their skin moisturized during pregnancy seem to develop fewer stretch marks.

An Expert's Opinion on

PREGNANCY AND BREAST SELF-EXAMS

During pregnancy you may notice that your breasts have become harder, with a thicker feeling, and possibly lumpy—all usually the result of growing milk ducts. Thus, you may be tempted to put off your monthly breast self-exams until after delivery. Doing so, however, would be a big mistake. According to breast expert Dr. Susan Love, pregnancy should never stop you from examining your breasts, particularly since high estrogen levels can cause any breast tumors that went unnoticed before to grow exceedingly fast now.

To help make breast exams easier, do them in the shower, putting lots of soap on your hands, which will make finding any lumps easier. (Experts say it's okay to soap up your nipples once a month when checking your breasts.) What should you be looking for? The same things as you did before pregnancy, says Love: "A distinct lump that feels different from the rest of your breast tissue." If the lump lasts for more than a week, she says, bring it to your doctor's attention. Sometimes breast lumps occurring during pregnancy can be the result of a blocked milk duct. When this is the case, says Love, it will likely feel more like a firm "wedge" than a lump, plus it is apt to disappear after massaging the breast or taking a warm shower.

Those that do occur are often less severe and more likely to disappear after baby is born. Moisturizing your breast skin may also keep you from developing an irritating nipple and breast itch, a common occurrence during pregnancy.

When choosing a breast moisturizer, look for a light, nongreasy, nonperfumed formula. If the consistency is very oily or thick, you could block natural breast secretions of colostrum—the premilk fluid that "tests" the efficiency of your milk ducts during pregnancy. Blocking this fluid release could lead to inflammation and ultimately infection in those ducts.

If a breast itch or inflammation does develop, talk to your doctor

Real Life

BREAST IMPLANTS AND PREGNANCY

Q: I just found out I'm pregnant. It's a bit of a surprise, and I'm very concerned because I have breast implants. I'm worried they will interfere with breast-feeding, but also that all the pressure associated with the natural increase in breast size during pregnancy will cause my implants to rupture—and I can't think of anything worse to happen during my pregnancy. Should I be worried?

A: Concerned, yes, but worried . . . most experts say no. Here's why: Assuming your implants were put in by a reputable surgeon, chances are very good that functional breast tissue was not affected. As long as the nerve and blood supply were left intact—which is highly likely—then you should have no problems breast-feeding. According to breast-feeding expert and instructor Anne Smith, while you may experience problems with your milk supply, including plugged ducts, these problems are easily corrected, and they also are common in women with no breast implants.

about the occasional use of hydrocortisone creams. Since these preparations contain potentially powerful steroids, don't use them without your doctor's okay.

In addition to stretch marks, some women also experience pronounced blue or even red veins on the surface of their breasts—some of which can take on an alarming, bulging appearance. While the condition may look scary, generally it is the result of increased circulation that causes vessels close to the skin to fill to capacity. If the sight of bluish veins really bothers you—particularly when wearing a swimsuit or camisole top—try one of the cosmetic concealers explored in Chapter 3, particularly the waterproof Dermablend, which offers great coverage that lasts until you take it off.

In terms of rupture, California plastic surgeon Dr. Scott R. Miller reports that there should be no pregnancy-related complications that can increase health risks over and above what they normally are for any woman with implants, including a natural risk of rupture. Your increasing breast size during pregnancy, however, should not increase that risk or affect your implant. But what if a rupture does occur? As long as your implants are saline—soft silicone shells filled with harmless saltwater—it should pose no risk to your baby. It also should not interfere with breast milk.

If your implants are filled with silicone gel, safety issues are slightly less clear. Studies show there is about 1.5 percent chance of leakage—and whether the silicone gets into your bloodstream or your milk supply depends on many factors, including the size of the silicone molecules, how much makes its way to the bloodstream, and the ability of the particular silicone to bind to human proteins. So, while you shouldn't worry just because you have implants, if yours do happen to rupture, you should seek medical advice as soon as possible.

One bit of good news: Dr. Miller suggests that women who have breast implants before pregnancy often have an easier time retaining the shape of their breasts after pregnancy.

PREPARING YOUR BREASTS FOR BREAST-FEEDING: WHAT TO DO NOW

In the not-too-distant past, many doctors routinely suggested that women prepare their breasts for breast-feeding by twisting, rolling, and pulling on the nipples, beginning somewhere in the third trimester. Even today some doctors still subscribe to this preparatory treatment. The logic is that manipulating the nipples and the skin around them reduces the irritation and inflammation that some women experience when breast-feeding begins. While it *may* help, there is little in the way of medical proof that it makes any significant difference, since, once breast-feeding begins, your nipples adjust fairly quickly.

One reason **not** to try third-trimester nipple stimulation: It could increase your risk of an early delivery. Indeed, when nipples are stimulated the hormone oxytocin is released, which in turn causes uterine contractions, sometimes strong enough to induce labor. If you are already at risk for premature labor—if you are carrying more than one baby, for example, if you are diagnosed with a weak or incompetent cervix, or if you have had premature labor in the past—then nipple manipulation is not for you, so do check with your doctor before engaging in this activity.

If, however, you suffer from inverted nipples (if they respond to squeezing by moving inward and going flat), there are steps you can take prior to giving birth that might make breast-feeding easier. Among the best things you can do is to begin wearing breast shields sometime in your third trimester. These are small, hard, rounded "shells" with a hole in the middle. You slip the shield inside your bra and center the hole on your nipple. The pressure from your breast pushing against the shield will force your nipples through the holes, helping them to become more erect—which can make it easier for your baby to latch on and begin breast-feeding. Breast shields are sold in most maternity-wear shops.

For more information on what to expect from your breasts after your baby is born, check out Chapter 12.

Pregnancy and Your Intimate Hygiene: What You Need to Know

Whether or not you develop any specific V zone problems during pregnancy, there are certain "normal" conditions that are going to require some extra care. I'm speaking about your intimate hygiene—and the fact that not all of your previous personal grooming routines will work as well, or be as safe, as they were before pregnancy.

In fact, because of the extra discharge that comes with pregnancy, as well as an increase in sweat and continence problems, many women complain that their normal intimate hygiene practices no longer seem adequate. In fact, doctors report that one of the most common questions they hear is whether a douche can help. The answer, say experts, is a resounding no. Unless you have a specific infection that requires a medicated douche, not only is douching unnecessary, it's unhealthy, particularly during pregnancy. Because it can alter the natural acid balance in your vagina, douching can increase your risk of infection—which in turn may threaten your pregnancy. It can also increase irritation in your vaginal tissues, which may be more tender at this time. Although it's rare, douching can also introduce air into your vagina, resulting in serious complications for you and your baby.

If you're thinking that intimate deodorants may be your answer, well, think again. Because they can contain many chemicals, most doctors are wary of their use during pregnancy. Since the mucous membranes inside your vagina are much like sponges, soaking up anything they come in contact with and transporting it directly into your bloodstream, chemicals that are applied directly to your V zone could, at least theoretically, reach your baby. While no studies have been done specifically to show if these products can cross the placenta or if they can cause harm to you or your baby, most doctors agree that the fewer chemicals you use on your body during pregnancy, the less you have to worry that a problem might occur.

Your best hygiene bet is to simply wash your V zone with warm water—no soap. Then use cornstarch-based powder (no talc) to absorb perspiration and wetness. Not only does cornstarch absorb better, it has none of the suspected links to ovarian disease that some studies have shown can be associated with heavy use of talcum powder. Good product choices include Johnson & Johnson Baby Powder Cornstarch Formula, Burt's Bees Cornstarch Dusting Powder, or Vagisil Powder with Double Odor Protection, which is made with cornstarch and is 100 percent talc free.

If you just don't feel clean unless you use a cleanser, try one specifically for the vagina, such as Vagisil's Hypoallergenic Cleansing Foam. Although the manufacturer says it's safe for use during pregnancy, do get your obstetrician's okay before trying this or any intimate care product.

PREGNANCY AND THE V ZONE ITCH: WHAT YOU CAN DO

As your pregnancy progresses, you may find you are plagued with a persistent V zone itch—a problem that can grow worse if you are pregnant during the summer months. While sometimes itching can be a sign of in-

Mother *Nature* Knows Best

TRY SEX FOR YOUR VAGINAL ITCH!

Well, maybe your mom wouldn't make the suggestion, but Mother Nature tells us that often sex can be among the best remedies for a non-infectious vaginal itch occurring during pregnancy—or any time. The reason has to do with semen ejaculate, which is usually highly acidic. The extra acid in your vagina may help restore a proper acid-alkaline balance, which in turn might relieve your itch.

fection, more often it is simply the result of raging hormones. As estrogen and progesterone climb, they can slightly alter the natural chemical balance inside your vagina, making the skin in and around your vulva itch.

In many instances, the problem will resolve without treatment. If it doesn't, talk to your doctor about the use of over-the-counter anti-itch creams formulated specifically for your pregnant V zone. Among those most recommended include Vagisil Feminine Itch Cream and Gynecort Anti-Itch Creme, which are both reported to be safe to use during pregnancy. If you want to take the all-natural approach, try a simple cold compress soaked in a solution of 1 cup of water mixed with several teaspoons of baking soda. Or soak a tea bag in warm water, cool it in the fridge, and apply it directly to the area of your vagina that is itching.

For some pregnant women, a vaginal itch takes a backseat to an itchy rectum, a problem doctors call pruritus ani. What can help is a bit of petroleum jelly. Apply it directly on your itchy skin, and wait several minutes before pulling up your panties. Since petroleum jelly can stain, you can place an ultra-thin menstrual pad near the back of your panties to absorb the excess grease.

If your chubby pregnant thighs or bulging belly are causing a chafing between your legs or under your tummy, make certain to rinse your skin throughly after a bath or shower and dry off completely. Soap residues, or even dampness, can exacerbate skin irritation and destroy some of the natural oil secretions that help keep skin lubricated and friction free.

BODY HAIR REMOVAL AND PREGNANCY:
WHAT'S SAFE, WHAT'S NOT

If you normally wax, bleach, or chemically remove hair from your V zone, thighs, legs, or underarms, you may be wondering if it's safe to continue this practice during pregnancy. Tending to body hair removal may be especially important if you are pregnant during summer months, when more of you is on display.

Certainly, the old standby method is to simply shave excess hair using an electric or disposable hand razor. Though it may not be what you are used to, it involves no chemicals and no stress to your skin, so it would be your safest choice. You can also try waxing, which doctors also say is safe. However, be aware that your genital area will be ultrasensitive during pregnancy, so it may hurt more, and you are more likely to see breakage of small blood vessels under the skin in the area where you are waxed.

While there are virtually no studies to indicate that bleaching body hair would be a problem during pregnancy, that doesn't automatically mean the process is safe. It could simply mean that it hasn't been adequately studied. While most experts say to avoid bleaching, epidemiologist Christina Chambers from the California Teratogenic Information Service says if you do bleach body hair, minimize risks by first rinsing skin in cold water (to close down pores) and work in a well-ventilated room.

Experts say the same advice applies if you are using a chemical depilatory—a liquid hair remover that works below the surface of the skin to dissolve hair at its roots. Although there are no studies to indicate that using these products during pregnancy can cause a problem, again, doctors say this could be because the compounds have not been adequately studied. If you want to use a chemical depilatory during pregnancy, be certain to check with your doctor, and do bring the product to your prenatal appointment so he or she can check the ingredients.

PERSPIRATION AND PREGNANCY:
WHAT YOU CAN DO

High levels of the hormone progesterone combined with increased circulation means your pregnant body is running hotter than normal. As a result, you may find you are perspiring more, particularly during physical activity. In addition, the extra weight of your baby requires much more effort to move your body, so you may also find yourself perspiring sooner than you normally would when doing any form of exercise, or even just walking.

While sweating may not feel comfortable, it does help to cool your body down whenever overheating occurs—something that's essential to your baby's health. Remember, when you get hot, your baby gets hot too—only there is no way for heat to immediately escape in the uterus! Nonetheless, it's *also* important that you remain comfortable during your pregnancy, particularly if you are working outside the home.

To help you stay cooler and drier, do what you do when you are not pregnant: Wear light clothing, in layers, and remove them as soon as you begin to feel warm. When exercising, skip the warm nylon and spandex clothing—it's hot and restrictive—and instead wear woven fabric that lets your skin breathe and allows body heat to escape.

Doctors suggest you avoid the use of heavy antiperspirants—the kind that stop sweat. While you can use deodorant products that help control the bacteria that contributes to perspiration odors, generally, sweating is a good thing during pregnancy, something you don't want to inhibit. You might want to look into purchasing a "natural" deodorant—either the rock crystal stones or products such as Orjene's Natural Deodorants, in chamomile or citrus scents, or Tom's of Maine Natural Deodorant Soap.

What can also help are quick but frequent lukewarm showers or baths to help keep sweat off your body. Afterward, dust off with a cornstarch-based powder, which can absorb up to twenty-five times more wetness than ordinary talc. Be certain to powder those areas where skin touches skin—such as under the breasts, just under your growing belly, and between your thighs. Doing so will help you avoid chafing, heat rash, and irritation.

To cool down and deal with excess perspiration in work or social situations, carry baby wipes in your purse. If you duck into the ladies' room and give your underarms a quick swipe, you'll be odor free and feel just-showered fresh.

YOUR PERSONAL PREGNANCY SPA

Although soaking in a relaxing warm tub can be an excellent way to cleanse your body, during pregnancy it can do double duty by also helping to relieve your stress. However, do note that it is important to monitor the temperature of your bathwater during pregnancy. When bathwater is too hot, it will not only dry out your pregnant skin, it might also harm your baby, increasing the risk of birth defects or miscarriage. Ideally, water that is around 100 degrees is best suited for the pregnant body. However, if you just can't live without at least an occasional steamy soak, the American College of Obstetricians and Gynecologists says bathwater can go as high as 102 degrees—but at that temperature, you shouldn't spend more than ten minutes in the tub. Additionally, don't add more hot water after you've been bathing for a while unless you use a bath thermometer, even if you think the water is starting to cool. The reason: As your body becomes used to the warmer water, you lose some sensitivity to heat, so you may not realize how hot your bath actually is.

If you want to enjoy a fragrant as well as a relaxing bath, consider adding fruits, flowers, or other natural ingredients to your tub water. Not only can this pamper your skin, it can also enliven your senses and offer some true therapeutic effects. While you can add almost any natural ingredient to your bath, here are a few secret favorites from spas around the world.

- Milk—powdered or fresh. Add as much as you like for silky, smooth skin.

- Pineapple. Contains bromelain, a natural enzyme that can improve skin tone. Squeeze fresh pineapple juice or use fresh frozen or canned juice, about ½ cup for each bath.

- Honey. A few tablespoons under running water will give your bath a sensuous fragrance. Honey also has disinfectant properties and can help soothe body acne.

- Oranges, lemons, and limes. Grate the rinds and add them to your bath; use slices of lemon to soothe rough knees, heels, and elbows.

- Vanilla extract. A few drops in your tub will relax your body and your mind.

For skin that is ultra-dry:

- Add 1 tablespoon of avocado, sesame, or wheat germ oil to a tubful of water.

For skin that is moderately dry:

- Add 1 tablespoon of almond, apricot, or vitamin E oil to a tubful of water.

For skin that is oily but lacking moisture:

- Add 1 teaspoon of calendula or safflower oil to a tubful of water.

When skin is itchy, red, inflamed, or irritated, you can add a handful or two of oatmeal to your bath. But if getting your spa ingredients from the kitchen cabinet takes away some of the glamour of your pampering ritual, then try Aveeno soothing Bath Treatment with 100 Percent Natural Colloidal Oatmeal, or the Baby Bee Buttermilk Bath from Burt's Bees to soothe irritated skin.

Your Intimate Health: A Final Word

Although your breasts and your V zone make up a highly resilient and sophisticated system that is developed specifically to withstand the rigors of pregnancy and childbirth, that doesn't mean you won't benefit from even just a little pampering care. If you work outside the home, keep a supply of hygiene products with you or at the office—including incontinence pads, breast pads, a container of cornstarch powder, a soft cleansing cloth, baby wipes, and some extra underwear—to help you feel fresher and more confident throughout your day.

If you should develop any unusual breast or V zone problems during pregnancy, check with your doctor right away. Catching problems early can minimize the threat of infection and help keep you and your baby safer and more comfortable throughout all three trimesters.

The Glow Factor

*Skin Care Secrets Every Pregnant Woman
Needs to Know*

I t's not just a myth, it's rooted in scientific fact: There *is* a special
"glow" that comes with being pregnant. While some say it's the sheer
joy of impending motherhood that lights up a woman's face, doctors take a bit more scientific slant, pointing instead to the increased circulation and other physiologic events of pregnancy as the source of that
rosy glow. And, in fact, when your pregnancy and your hormones are
humming along at a perfect pace, that's precisely what you *will* experience.

Unfortunately, this isn't always the case. As your hormones begin to
ebb and flow, climbing up, falling back, and generally tripping over each
other in a race to get your body ready for baby, you can begin experiencing many of the same skin problems that occur just prior to a monthly
menstrual cycle—a time when reproductive hormones also seem to take
on a life of their own.

But unlike during your monthly cycle, when the arrival of your period brings a quick halt to any temporary skin flare-ups, in pregnancy
those hormones continue to rage, sometimes taking weeks or even

months to stabilize. In the process, your skin—including not only your face but your entire body—can continue to react. Excess oiliness; breakouts; parched and dry patches; excessive sensitivity to cleansers, creams, soaps, and gels; makeup that just doesn't look right anymore; and, for many, a "pregnancy mask" that causes splotchy discolorations on your cheeks, your nose, even your body are just some of the problems that you may have already begun to encounter. Complicating things further, concern for your baby may cause you to be reluctant to use many of the chemical products, skin treatments, or even cosmetics that you relied on in the past to pull you through. In fact, some of these products—including a variety of acne medications—may not be safe to use during pregnancy at all.

Moreover, just as you think you have your skin back under control, you enter a new trimester and a whole *new* series of complexion problems develop. Stretch marks, skin tags, moles, and a dry itchy rash that can drive you to distraction; any or all can come together to make your pregnancy more uncomfortable than it has to be. Your concerns may, in fact, take on an even greater importance if you are a working mother-to-be and must continue to maintain a polished and professional appearance throughout your pregnancy.

But if having a baby is starting to sound less and less like something you are going to enjoy, don't despair. While there will be some bumps along the road, the important thing to remember is that there are an abundance of new ways to cope with even the most frustrating of these problems, keeping you looking and feeling better than you ever have before. In fact, some of what you might learn about yourself and your body while you are pregnant can continue to serve you well long after your baby is born.

The end result: a pregnancy during which you not only glow but you feel as terrific as you look!

The Five Most Common Pregnancy Skin Problems and How to Beat Them

PROBLEM #1: THE PREGNANCY MASK

Among the most common skin conditions associated with pregnancy is known as chloasma or sometimes melasma. But you probably know it as the pregnancy mask—named for the placement of the brown-hued pigmentation that usually occurs in the center of the face, often across the cheeks and bridge of the nose. According to the American Academy of Dermatology, melasma can affect up to 70 percent of all pregnant women to varying degrees.

But where does pregnancy mask come from? Just underneath the top layer of your skin (called the epidermis) lies a layer of cells known as melanocytes. When stimulated by any number of factors, including the sun, melanocytes produce melanin—the biochemical that helps you achieve your summer tan. But sun isn't the only factor responsible for melanocytes. Pregnancy hormones cause an increase in levels of a natural body chemical known as MSH—short for melanocyte-stimulating hormone. As levels of MSH increase, melanocytes get the signal to begin producing more pigment.

Unfortunately, since cell stimulation occurs in just certain areas of the body, you won't end up with a pregnancy "tan" but instead a pregnancy "mask." Because women with darker complexions naturally harbor more melanocytes, they often experience a more intense pregnancy mask—with brunettes generally more susceptible than blondes. Regardless of your hair color, however, you may also find darker areas of pigmentation on and around your nipples and between your thighs. You may also develop a line down the center of your tummy known as the *linea nigra,* or "line of pregnancy"—a skin discoloration that occurs as your belly starts to really grow.

PREVENTING PREGNANCY MASK: WHAT REALLY WORKS

While there is no foolproof way to prevent a pregnancy mask from forming, you can reduce your risks by making certain you get adequate amounts of the B vitamin *folic acid.* Studies show that this same nutrient

Real Life

SUNSCREEN, FOUNDATION, AND
PREGNANCY MASK

Q: My foundation contains a sunscreen with an SPF of 15. Will that be enough protection for me, or will I still need a sunscreen product to protect against pregnancy mask?

A: If you're going to be out of doors for two hours or less, then, yes, your foundation probably will be sufficient. However, if you plan to spend the day outdoors, or if you are in and out a number of times throughout the day, foundation might not do the job. In fact, studies show that normal facial movements, such as smiling or frowning, can cause foundation to slip and slide, shifting and wearing off rapidly—a problem that is exacerbated if your skin is the least bit oily. In a study published in the *Journal of the American Academy of Dermatology*, doctors reported testing a variety of foundation types, including lotions, liquids, and cream/powder combinations, on a variety of women with dry, oily, and normal and combination skin types. Using a medical-grade camera, they recorded how the products fared on the skin.

The result: After just two hours, the camera revealed makeup shifted from the surface of the skin into the fine lines and crevices. Those with oily skin experienced the fastest "slide." The cream/powder foundation settled in lines the most *and* the most quickly on all skin types.

Eventually, nearly all the makeup moved from the top layer of the skin deep into tiny hair follicles and pores, leaving the face bare and prone to sun exposure. To help ensure this doesn't happen to you, and to reduce your risk of pregnancy mask, always apply a sunscreen under your foundation.

that helps protect your baby against birth defects may also help *you* avoid pregnancy mask. The recommended dosage of folic acid during pregnancy is 400 micrograms daily. (See Chapter 6.)

Because the sun encourages the production of melanin in the skin, wearing a sunscreen with an SPF (sun protection factor) of 15 any time you are out of doors in daylight hours, winter *or* summer, can also help. Sunscreen products doctors frequently suggest for use during pregnancy include those that feature transparent zinc oxide, micronized zinc oxide, and titanium dioxide as their key ingredients. Because they lie on top of the skin and don't penetrate deeper layers, they aren't absorbed into your body or by your baby, so they are considered ultra safe to use during pregnancy.

One caveat: Because these ingredients can be sticky and thick, they may be harder to apply. For easier coverage, look for products that blend zinc oxide into a lotion formula, such as Belli Cosmetics Anti Chloasma Sunscreen with SPF 25.

The Great Cover-up: Hiding Your Pregnancy Mask

If, despite your best efforts, you still develop a pregnancy mask, fear not: It's likely to fade soon after you deliver. In the meantime, a few simple cosmetics can rescue your complexion with hardly any effort at all.

If your pregnancy mask is light to medium in color, you may need nothing more than a highly pigmented foundation in a color that matches your natural skin tone. If the product is saturated with color, you get a lot of coverage without having to use a lot of product. You can tell if a product has a lot of pigment by testing the opacity on the back of your hand. If it's able to cover the vein discolorations we all have, as well as hide pores, then it's likely to cover a pregnancy mask. Choosing a stick or cream foundation instead of a liquid can be a plus, since coverage tends to be more complete. Products that fit this description include Smashbox Cosmetics Foundation Stick, Make Up Forever's Pan Stick, Max Factor Pan Stick, or Maybelline Express 3 in 1 Cream Stick.

What can also help is choosing a shade that is closest to your natural skin color. "If you select a very light shade, you're not going to get better coverage, and you may only draw more attention to the mask because you're highlighting that area," says makeup artist Holly Stougard-Mordini, vice president of Smashbox Cosmetics.

But if your pregnancy mask is very dark, then a super-industrial-strength undereye concealer with heavily pigmented color may be your best bet. One tip when applying any concealer—whether you are pregnant or not—is to put on a good moisturizer first or prime your skin using an under-makeup base. Either one will help the concealer go on more smoothly, plus give you good coverage with minimal product. A good concealer choice is Camouflage by Dermacolor, a staple for generations of Hollywood makeup artists, not only because it covers completely, but because it sets without the need for powder. So, it won't leave a dry or cakey look on the skin. Other good choices include Adrienne Arpel's Industrial Strength Concealer or Dermablend's Quick Fix compact cover cream or Cover Cream Corrective Duo.

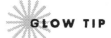 **GLOW TIP**

Choosing the Perfect Concealer

As good as a great concealer can be, a bad one can be a beauty disaster, creating more flaws than it covers. To find the perfect product for you, try these tips:

- Stay away from concealers that are white, chalky, pink toned, very greasy, or very dry to the touch.

- Look for concealers that are smooth, creamy in texture, yellow toned, and blend easily into your skin.

If you have the right concealer, you'll know it—because you'll look better the instant you put it on. If you don't, then either the color or the product is wrong for you.

Bobbi Brown, celebrity makeup artist, Bobbi Brown Cosmetics

WHEN YOUR PREGNANCY MASK DOESN'T DISAPPEAR: WHAT TO DO

For most women, a pregnancy mask, along with discolorations on the thighs and the stomach, will disappear shortly after giving birth—usually within two months. But when this isn't the case, a variety of treatments can help. Among the newest involves a combination of Retin A—an acid lotion that peels away top layers of dead skin cells—coupled with hydroquinone, a bleaching agent for the skin. Because both are harsh treatments, you should never use these products during pregnancy or attempt these procedures on your own after giving birth; you will definitely need the help of a dermatologist for safe and effective care.

A slightly different twist on the formula is a prescription topical cream called Tri-Luma. This combines the ingredients fluocinolone acetonide (0.01 percent) with hydroquinone (4 percent) and tretinoin (0.05 percent). Because safety profiles have not been established for use in pregnancy or while breast-feeding, doctors also suggest waiting until after your baby is born and breast-feeding is completed before considering this treatment.

You can also talk to your doctor about a facial-resurfacing treatment like laser dermabrasion. Here a light source emanating from a tiny laser beam lightly "burns" off the top layer of skin cells holding the pigmented mask. Because the treatment can be tricky when facial color is uneven, you'll need a well-schooled professional, preferably a board-certified dermatologist with experience in laser resurfacing. To find a doctor in your area, contact the American Society of Dermatologic Surgery (www.asds-net.org) at 847-956-0900 or e-mail them at info@aboutskin surgery.com.

By the way, if you're thinking that you'd like to try a laser treatment *during* pregnancy, most doctors are against the idea. Studies show that during pregnancy the mask has a tendency to return after treatment—so you may not see relief for very long.

PROBLEM #2: CAUGHT IN THE WEB OF SPIDER VEINS

Medically they're known as telangiectasis, but mostly we know them as spider veins, the reddish-blue lines resembling the tentacles of a spider that can develop just below the surface of the skin. While they most often occur on the legs and stomach, some women can develop them on the face.

They are caused by an increase in blood volume that occurs as your pregnancy progresses. This results in additional pressure inside your veins, which, in turn, can cause tiny capillaries lying just under the surface of the skin to rupture and leak. When they do, the fine red- or blue-tinged lines appear. Formation usually peaks in the second trimester, when blood volume is highest, so it's not likely they will get any worse than what you see at this time. And, most often they will disappear shortly after delivery, or sometimes even during the third trimester. In the meantime, you can cover up spider veins using the same concealing techniques that work for pregnancy mask.

If, however, you're looking to treat or even prevent spider veins from developing, many women report success with vitamin K cream, which some research shows may penetrate the skin and clot the blood that's leaking from the capillaries just under the surface. In order to work, however, the cream must contain at least 5 percent vitamin K, and it must be applied at least twice daily. If you already have spider veins, it could take four weeks or more to see any significant difference in your skin. Because vitamin K has blood-clotting properties, do mention your interest in these creams to your obstetrician and get his or her okay before you try them.

Natural medicine experts also recommend arnica gel to reduce the redness in spider veins. Long used by plastic surgeons to reduce bruising after face-lifts, arnica contains properties that constrict blood vessels and encourage healing. Again, talk to your obstetrician first—particularly if you are anticipating the need for a cesarean section birth.

If your spider veins don't disappear after pregnancy—the case for up to 25 percent of women—laser therapy can help seal the leaks in your facial capillaries and eliminate the discoloration.

PROBLEM #3: OILY SKIN AND PREGNANCY ACNE

For many women, the high hormone levels of pregnancy can have a beneficial effect on acne, allowing their skin to look and feel smoother and more radiant than ever before. For some, however, the exact opposite can be true. For these women, fluctuating levels of both estrogen and progesterone can make acne worse.

If your skin normally breaks out during your period, it might be worse during early pregnancy, when your hormones are fluctuating sim-

Real Life

THE "KISS" MOLE

Q: I am in my second month of pregnancy and seem to be growing what my husband has lovingly nicknamed "kiss moles," because he says they look like tiny red kisses. In reality, they are small, red, semisolid bumps that look a lot like they could be filled with blood. They are on my face and now starting on my arms. My OB said they are nothing to worry about but didn't explain further. I'm always afraid they'll start to bleed. What are they, and should they be removed?

A: This problem matches the description of a spider hemangioma—another variation of the spider vein. These are tightly wound balls of tiny vessels that grow into the bright red bumps you describe, but they are not likely to bleed. Often pregnant women develop these growths—sometimes just a few, sometimes hundreds all over their body. And they can grow bigger as pregnancy progresses. While no one is certain how or why they occur, they have been linked to increased estrogen production. As hormone levels climb, blood vessels can be stimulated to the point where the tiny red "kiss moles" you describe develop.

Pregnancy hormones can also encourage the growth of skin tags, warts, and moles, and those that are present before pregnancy may grow after you conceive. While nearly all these growths are harmless, it's important to bring *any* skin changes to your doctor's attention during your regular prenatal visits. You will also want to see your dermatologist *after* baby is born to discuss any changes that might occur in tags or moles. Hormones going up and down in the postpartum period can sometimes initiate harmful growths, so it's important to keep your eye on your skin and compare it often to how it looked prior to pregnancy. If the growths that occur during pregnancy don't disappear after delivery, most can be safely removed via laser therapy.

ilarly to when you are menstruating each month. Even women who never had a breakout before may develop acne for the first time during pregnancy—thanks to those bouncing hormones. Indeed, as levels of estrogen and progesterone climb, they stimulate oil production. When oil is produced faster than it can exit your pores, a kind of "biological traffic jam" occurs; oil and other cellular debris begin sticking together, causing a blockage in the pathway that leads to your pores. The more oil that is produced, the bigger the blockage can get, until finally inflammation sets in. When this occurs, bacteria are released into the mix, which eventually cause a pimple to develop. The longer your pores remained blocked, the greater the likelihood that acne will occur.

ACNE TREATMENTS: WHAT'S SAFE, WHAT'S NOT

Whether you have had acne in the past or just suffered an occasional breakout, you probably know there is certainly no shortage of treatments from which to choose. Once pregnancy enters the equation, however, the list grows somewhat shorter. At least one popular prescription acne drug, an oral retinoid treatment known as isotretinoin (Accutane, Roaccutane), was proven so potentially harmful to baby that today doctors won't even prescribe it unless a woman is using birth control. Use during pregnancy is obviously out of the question.

Another popular treatment option includes derivatives of isotretinoin—topical medications such as Retin A. But now these are also under fire. While no prospective studies have shown they increase the risk of birth defects, anecdotal stories and some medical case reports have, leading many doctors to place this medication on the "no" list during pregnancy. Another common acne drug, the broad-spectrum antibiotic tetracycline, has been linked to dental-related birth defects, so it's not commonly recommended during pregnancy either.

What Do Doctors Say Is Safe to Try?

- Topical or oral forms of the antibiotic erythromycin

- Topical forms of the antibiotic clindamycin (Cleocin)

- Topical azelaic acid (Azelex)

- Topical sodium sulfacetamide

Also Safe to Use in Moderation (for spot treatments or occasional use)

- Products containing the ingredients salicylic acid or benzoyl peroxide

- Adaptalene, a topical derivative of vitamin A used in Differin Gel

Important note: Never use any acne treatment without checking with your obstetrician. If you regularly see a dermatologist, make certain she or he knows you are pregnant. Never take any medication that was prescribed to you prior to conception after you become pregnant, unless your doctor advises you to do so.

STOPPING A BREAKOUT BEFORE IT STARTS: WHAT YOU CAN DO

One of the best ways to avoid an acne breakout—during pregnancy or any time—is to keep the passageways between your oil glands and your pores free and clear. One of the best ways to do that is via the use of a skin exfoliator—a cream that removes dead skin cells from the top layer of your complexion, thereby helping to keep pores open. Among the most popular forms of exfoliation are creams containing alpha hydroxy acids (AHAs)—fruit acids and natural sugars that help dislodge the dead skin cells that can block pores.

Although there are no studies to prove either the safety or the dangers of alpha hydroxy acid use in pregnancy, because they can penetrate into the deeper layers of skin, some physicians are hesitant to recommend them. Others, however, feel that as long as your product contains a low percentage of AHAs—5 percent or less—then it's not likely to cause any danger to your baby. So if you want to try these products, don't shop in beauty supply houses that supply professional-grade AHAs with a high acid content. Instead, seek out consumer products that keep AHA content low. Then use the products sparingly—only where you really need them. Good examples of mild AHA products include Pond's Age Defying Lotion for Delicate Skin, Avon's Anew All-in-One Perfecting Lotion, and Avon All-in-One Perfecting Creme.

Real Life

NATURAL ACNE BUSTERS

To safely loosen dead skin cells and help create that pregnancy glow, the editors of *Natural Health* magazine offer the following recipe for cleaner, healthier skin.

What You Need: In a food processor, grind ¼ cup of rolled oats into a finely milled powder. Combine with 1 to 2 tablespoons of water, and mix until it's the consistency of peanut butter.

What to Do: Apply to the skin, working the paste in small circles for about five minutes. Be sure to concentrate on extra-oily areas, such as the tops of the cheeks, sides of the nose, chin, and forehead. Do, however, avoid your delicate eye area. Rinse with warm water and pat dry.

How It Helps: The oats provide the natural exfoliation that removes dead cells safely, without chemicals.

A second highly effective natural treatment involves the topical application of a plant-based preparation known as tea tree oil—a natural antiseptic that has been used in Europe and China for centuries to control the growth of bacteria.

To Use: Dip a clean cotton swab into undiluted tea tree oil, and then lightly dab the areas where your breakouts are occurring. Used once or twice daily, it can help reduce both inflammation and the risk of infection.

If you'd like to skip the use of AHAs altogether, you can still exfoliate with a skin "scrub"—products containing tiny bits of crushed almond, walnuts, or apricot seeds used to mechanically lift up and remove layers of dead skin cells on the surface of your face. Used two to three times weekly, they can help keep acne at bay, and the extra circulation can help increase blood flow to the face and encourage that rosy glow. Do not, however, use a scrub on skin that is inflamed or irritated.

GLOW TIP

Hide It, Hide It, Hide It!

If, despite your best efforts, pregnancy breakouts are something you just can't avoid, not to fret—with the right technique you can cover almost any blemish and make it all but disappear. Try this technique:

1. Apply foundation as usual.

2. Dip a concealer brush into a cream or stick foundation (liquid won't give you enough coverage) in a shade that matches your face exactly.

3. Gently paint the foundation over the blemish and blend—don't rub—with your fingertip.

4. Place a small amount of powder on a puff and lock the coverage in place.

Bobbi Brown, celebrity makeup artist, Bobbi Brown Cosmetics

PROBLEM #4: DESERT-DRY PREGNANCY SKIN

As your baby grows, his or her need for fluid dramatically increases. In an effort to meet those needs, beginning somewhere around the second trimester, water is pulled from all your cells—including those in your skin. Not surprisingly, even if you had oily skin at the start of your pregnancy, you may find you have dry, flaking skin by the time you reach your third trimester. If you started your pregnancy with a normal or especially an arid complexion, dryness and flaking on your face and on your body can begin appearing even sooner—sometimes at the start of your second trimester.

As is the case when you *aren't* pregnant, the best defense against dry skin is to keep it hydrated by drinking at least eight cups of water a day. This is in addition to any other juices, teas, or beverages you consume. Simply put, the more water you drink, the less your baby's needs will tug on your cell supply and the less will be pulled from your skin. And that means more hydrated, healthier skin, not only on your face but on your entire body. Of course, it also means a few extra trips to the bathroom—but hey, isn't great skin worth it?

Next in line is your choice of cleansers—and in this instance what you *don't* use may be more important that what you do. If your skin is very dry, avoid soap completely. Most are extremely alkaline, meaning they can strip your skin of natural oils. If your skin is already dry, this can cause major problems. However, a liquid, nonsoap cleanser or a cleansing cream made for the face can gently dissolve impurities without disrupting your natural oil or acid balance. In addition, if you have dry skin, always wash your face with your fingers, not a washcloth and never a loofah. You should also avoid alcohol-based toners and instead opt for a witch hazel–based product. Or avoid the toner altogether.

When it comes to choosing a body cleanser, look for bar soaps labeled "super fatty," which are enriched with natural oils such as coconut, jojoba, or vitamin E. These ingredients will nourish skin and prevent dryness. For ultra-sensitive skin choose a glycerin soap, which has natural moisturizing properties and won't strip natural oils from the skin.

If you prefer a bath gel to soap, the same advice applies. Seek out those with the most natural skin-pampering ingredients, including calendula (made from marigolds), lavender and chamomile flowers, honey (a natural disinfectant and skin humidifier), and peach, apricot kernel, or jojoba oils (extremely moisturizing). Ideally, these ingredients should be listed among the first few compounds in your soap or washing gel. Other options include Belli Cosmetics Comfort Cleansing Body Wash and Oil of Olay's Complete Body Wash for Sensitive Skin, both of which offer among the purest ingredients available.

Finally, whether using a bath gel or a bar soap, try not to regularly suds your breasts—doing so can further dry the natural oils on the surface of your skin that will protect your nipples from pregnancy-induced inflammation. In addition, make certain to rinse your breasts with clear water at the end of your bath, being certain to remove any soap residue.

Whenever possible, avoid all cleansing products that are heavy on fragrance. Not only will perfumes irritate dry skin, they are also the leading cause of allergic reactions. You should also skip using very hot water, sticking instead to lukewarm or cool rinses. Most important is to always use a moisturizer after washing either your face or body.

What you want to avoid completely, particularly on your face, are harsh skin exfoliants, including high-potency AHAs and some mechanical scrubs, many of which can harm delicate, dry skin. Instead, wash away dead, dry skin cells with a product containing gentle cleansing "beads" instead of natural chunks of nuts or seeds found in many scrubs. Good product choices for the face or body include St. Ives Ultra Gentle Apricot Scrub for Sensitive Skin or the Principal Secret Exfoliating Scrub.

In addition, don't overlook the power of using products designed for *your baby* after birth. Generally speaking, any product that is safe to use on a baby's skin is also safe for Mom to use during or after pregnancy. If the moisturizing properties aren't quite enough, supplement by adding nature-based products such as Elaria's Shea Butter Body Cream or Avocado and Lemon Grass Body Cream—both are extra rich and creamy and loaded with natural oils, or try Serious Skin Care's line of olive oil–based products.

A Drink for Your Thirsty Skin: What Your Face and Body Really Need

Because a dry, arid complexion needs both oil *and* moisture, look for facial and body care products in a cream rather than lotion formulation—as well as those containing hyaluronic acid. This important ingredient works to bind water to the skin at a rate of up to 1,000 times its weight. You will also benefit from products that contain liposomes—small particles that encapsulate moisturizer, delivering the rejuvenating ingredients into the deeper layers of your skin, where dryness begins. When possible, also choose products that are alcohol free and fragrance free, and keep chemical preservatives to a minimum. What can also help: applying facial moisturizer on damp skin and then waiting a few minutes before putting on your makeup. Doing this can help lock moisture in and dryness out.

Adding actual moisture—as in water—to your face during the day can also keep skin moist and supple. One of the best ways is via an Evian Face Mister. Designed to spray in an ultra-fine mist that won't disturb makeup and is readily absorbed into the skin, French dermatologists often use this product to keep the skin on burn victims hydrated. In addition, Evian water contains a mineral composition like that of the human

An Expert's Opinion on

DRY SKIN AND YOUR PREGNANCY HEALTH

For most women, dry skin is nothing more than their complexion's cry for moisture. However, for some women it is a sign of a health problem that can affect their baby and their postpartum recovery. According to experts from Johns Hopkins Medical Center, dry skin can *sometimes* be a symptom of hypothyroidism (underactive thyroid), a problem that may appear for the first time during pregnancy.

If caught early on, hypothyroidism is no threat to you or your baby, and the medication used to treat it is extremely safe. The problem, however, can be difficult to detect, mostly because its other symptoms, such as fatigue, mood swings, constipation, and muscle aches, can be confused with normal pregnancy complaints.

To make diagnosis easier, bring any incidence of sudden and especially extreme dry skin to the attention of your obstetrician, and discuss the possibility of taking a simple blood test that measures levels of TSH (thyroid-stimulating hormone). If levels are low, medication can bring your body up to speed. Doing so may not only improve pregnancy health, it can also make rebounding after birth faster and easier. Even if you don't get tested during pregnancy, if your skin remains very dry and fatigue or depression continue after birth, do talk to your doctor about testing for TSH. (See Chapter 12 for additional information on thyroid disorders and postpartum recovery.)

body—meaning you are dousing your skin with the most natural and most compatible moisture source possible. You can also add water to your skin via a room humidifier, which can be particularly helpful if your home has dry heat in winter or air-conditioning in summer. By keeping the air around you moist (particularly while you sleep), you will keep both your facial complexion and your overall body complexion hydrated, thereby reducing your need for skin care products and dry skin treatments.

Mother *Nature* Knows Best

PEACHES-AND-CREAM PREGNANCY

Longing for that peaches-and-cream complexion? Try using . . . peaches and cream! To exfoliate dry skin with a mild natural formula, try this recipe from the editors of *SELF* magazine.

Peel and mash a ripe peach, and strain through a sieve or put in a mechanical juicer. Blend the juice with an equal part of heavy whipping cream, and massage into skin. Leave on for up to twenty minutes, then rinse with warm water. You can make it ahead, and refrigerate up to forty-eight hours before use. The gentle fruit acids in the peach and the lactic acid in the cream will remove dry flaky skin and help give you a natural glow!

If you're feeling a bit more adventurous or would like to expand your array of natural skin care treatments, you can use almost any flower or fruit to make a body care cream, often for just pennies per treatment. Here are a few more recipes collected from beauty experts and top spas around the world.

LUSCIOUS-SKIN STRAWBERRY MOISTURIZER

Mix together 2 tablespoons mashed, crushed strawberries with 1 tablespoon each of coconut oil and olive oil. Apply directly to face and body. You can store any leftover mixture in an airtight container in the

---

PROBLEM #5: STRETCH MARKS

Among the most common of all pregnancy-related body complexion problems are stretch marks—those deep red, sometimes blue lines that can develop, usually beginning somewhere around your second trimester—on your tummy, breast, midsection, and even thighs. In fact, they are so common, up to 90 percent of women have them to some degree. Medically known as *striae gravidarum,* they frequently begin around the navel and fan out over your abdomen in what a pregnant girlfriend now refers to as a her "personal beach ball" pattern.

But how and why do they occur? Skin is divided into several layers.

refrigerator for up to ten days. Beauty and natural health expert Tina Cassady, who developed this formulation, reminds us that just eight strawberries have the vitamin C power of a whole orange—and vitamin C is what provides the collagen that holds skin cells together.

SWEET SPOT HONEY MOISTURIZER

Mix 1 teaspoon honey with 1 teaspoon vegetable oil and 1 teaspoon lemon juice. Rub into hands, elbows, heels, and anywhere that feels dry. Leave on for ten minutes. Rinse off with water.

ROSY GLOW SKIN QUENCHER

Combine 2 parts rose water with 1 part glycerin. Blend well to lotion consistency. Apply as often as needed to ease dry skin.

BODY SOFT COCOA BUTTER SKIN SOOTHER

From *Natural Beauty* author Donna Marie: In a heat-proof container, combine about 20 grams of unscented cocoa butter with 18 grams each of extra-virgin olive oil, sesame oil, and avocado oil, and place in a saucepan of boiling water. Heat until cocoa butter melts into the oils. Remove from heat and stir well. Pour into a glass bottle with a tight cap. Use several drops at a time to moisturize skin. If mixture hardens, run the bottle under warm water until it liquefies.

In the center layer, known as the dermis, lie collagen and elastin fibers— the components that actually help give your skin its elastic quality. But when skin is stretched abnormally, as it is during pregnancy, collagen and elastin begin to break down. In an attempt to repair itself, additional collagen fibers are quickly produced. The appearance of those fibers just under the surface of the skin causes those brightly colored lines we know as stretch marks.

For some women, it is the look of stretch marks that is the most annoying. But for others, how their stomach looks takes a backseat to how it *feels*—specifically the itching, tingling, even burning sensation that can accompany stretch marks, particularly on the tummy and breasts.

According to Tulane University professor of dermatology Dr. Nia

Terezakis, like the stretch marks themselves, the itching and other sensory perceptions are the result of skin stretching and are nothing to be alarmed about. Usually, says Dr. Terezakis, these sensations dissipate around the fourth month, at least on the breasts, although in some women the belly may continue to itch throughout the pregnancy.

Most often, natural products like aloe vera gel can soothe the itch, while moisturizers can ease the dry skin. If, however, your belly itch is severe or accompanied by a rash or blisters, see your doctor right away, and check on other possible problems found later in this chapter.

PREVENTING STRETCH MARKS: WHAT YOU CAN DO

While the folklore on how to prevent stretch marks is practically a cottage industry, the reality is that only a few factors can influence whether you experience this problem.

First and foremost are heredity and ethnic background, both of which can be contributing factors. If you want to know if you might develop stretch marks, ask your mom if she had them during pregnancy. And, if you yourself had them in a previous pregnancy, you are more likely to get them when you get pregnant again. African American women are the least likely group to develop stretch marks, while natural blondes with light complexions are at greatest risk. Additionally, if you are a light-skinned woman, your stretch marks will likely take on a pinkish hue, while if you have a darker skin, they may appear in a slightly lighter shade of your natural skin tone.

The good news is there are also some factors related to stretch marks that you *can* control. So, even if you are prone to this problem, there are ways to decrease your risks—starting with watching your weight and keeping extra pounds under control. How can this help? When skin is forced to stretch too rapidly, the underlying dermal structure is affected, which in turn influences the development of stretch marks. And while it is imperative that you gain a healthy amount of weight during your pregnancy (and you'll learn more on how to gauge a healthy gain in Chapter 6), a slow and gradual gain is best—not only for your baby, but for your body.

Equally important is keeping your overall body complexion well hydrated, particularly your stomach and breasts. This is particularly important if you are gaining weight quickly. Because skin that is supple and soft has more elastic qualities, you are less likely to experience stretch marks if your skin is well moisturized.

While all of the products suggested in the section on dry skin can be a big help, it's also important to remember that the more a product is absorbed into the skin, the more likely it is that tiny capillaries, already dilated from pregnancy, can pick up ingredients, including chemicals and preservatives, and carry them into your bloodstream where eventually they can reach your baby. This can be especially important when you are using products on your belly. While the amount that you retain will be exceptionably small and not much cause for concern, whenever possible doctors recommend that during pregnancy you choose the purest, most natural skin care products possible, particularly for use on the skin of your stomach. One product that can give you all the moisturizing properties you need without any risks is cocoa butter. An all-natural fat derived from the cocoa bean, its superior moisturizing power is legendary, particularly among pregnant women. While there is no *scientific* evidence to show that it prevents stretch marks, many doctors recommend its use.

The key, of course, is to use as close to 100 percent *pure* cocoa butter as you can find. One option is to order a medical grade cocoa butter from your pharmacist. Or you can try Aura Cacia Cocoa Butter, which is 100 percent natural and extremely pure.

For those who already are experiencing the red and blue lines, it's not too late to lubricate. Stretched skin that is kept supple and soft is far more likely to return to normal once your pregnancy weight is lost. Any stretch marks you do experience are also likely to disappear on their own, usually beginning two weeks after you deliver, if you keep your stomach well moisturized during pregnancy.

BELLY CREAMS AND STRETCH MARKS: WHAT YOU NEED TO KNOW

As you shop for skin care products during pregnancy, you will no doubt come across a variety of items known as belly creams. Designed to deliver intense moisture to your stomach, some manufacturers even claim these creams can reduce the risk of both stretch marks and the "belly itch" that can develop when skin stretches excessively. Obviously, not all products do what they say—so the rule of thumb here is "buyer beware."

That said, there are some formulations that can accomplish quite a bit more than the ordinary moisturizer. One brand-new ingredient is the scientifically tested botanical known as darutoside. An extract of the plant *Siegesbeckia orientalis,* it has been clinically shown to stimulate wound healing and tissue regeneration, and to restore elasticity by promoting the production of collagen, which is what breaks down as stretch marks occur. While there are no studies to indicate that use during pregnancy will prevent stretch marks, research does show that if you apply this ingredient starting the minute your baby is born, you could help fade the ones that did develop in four weeks or less. Currently it is found in only one product: Belli Cosmetic's Stretch Mark Minimizing Cream.

Magia Bella's Ultra Sensitive Anti-Stretch Mark Concentrate contains a trademarked ingredient (Elastigen SG) that reportedly has been shown to build the connective skin tissue that breaks down as your tummy grows. It's designed to be used in the third trimester, when stretch marks hit their stride.

You can also help minimize the development of stretch marks by applying an opened vitamin E capsule directly to your belly. (Puncture the capsule with a pin and squirt the contents onto your skin.) It works well alone or particularly in combination with the herb go-to kola, which has been shown in laboratory tests to help reduce the formation of stretch marks. Often the combination can be found in skin care products sold in health food stores. Or you can purchase Belli's Elasticity Belli Oil, which combines vitamin E and go-to kola, along with emu oil (which helps promote skin cell healing), as well as lavender and sweet almond oils to soothe and calm the senses.

Although you should feel free to try any moisturizer (particularly pure cocoa butter), what you *don't* want to use are products that feel exceptionally heavy, greasy, or overly oily to the touch. Most often, they will lie on the surface of your skin and not penetrate into the deeper layers, where help is really needed. While products containing a large amount of mineral oil or petroleum jelly (first or second on the ingredient list) may help reduce itching on the surface of your belly, they may not penetrate deep enough to affect collagen production or do anything to minimize your stretch marks, during or after pregnancy.

Preventing Stretch Marks Naturally

If you let her, Mother Nature could be your skin's best ally. Some of the most skin-quenching products you can use are those you make yourself with ingredients that can be found right in your kitchen. What you can try:

- Add 2 tablespoons of honey to a warm bath to draw moisture to your skin. If you're a shower girl, use a plastic squeeze bottle of honey to drench your tummy. Let it remain while you continue your shower. Rinse it off right before you're done.

- Make your own all-natural cocoa butter emulsion by heating equal parts of grated cocoa butter and coconut oil (to make application easier) in a microwave until melted. Stir well, let cool, and apply generously on your tummy, hips, buttocks, breasts, and arms.

- Soak a clean white cloth in a small dish of warm milk, squeeze out, and apply the compress to your belly for up to fifteen minutes. Dip the cloth several times, and reapply as needed.

- In *Natural Body Basics—Making Your Own Cosmetics,* expert author Dorie Byers offers this recipe for homemade moisturizer:

  2 tablespoons shea butter (available at many health food stores)

  1 tablespoon apricot-kernel oil

  1 teaspoon avocado oil

  ½ teaspoon rose hip seed oil

  800 international units (IU) vitamin E

  ½ teaspoon rose water

  6 drops lavender essential oil

  In a double boiler, melt the shea butter. Add apricot and avocado oils and remove from heat. Add rose hip seed oil and vitamin E, and blend using a wire whisk. When mixture is almost cool (it will look like pudding that is starting to set), add rose water and lavender oil. Once cool, pour into a wide-mouth jar. Let set until hardened (it could take quite a while, depending on temperature and humidity). Apply liberally to your skin as needed. If you keep it in a cool dry place, it should last up to two weeks or longer. One word of caution: This mixture should have a pleasant scent. If you can smell the oils when you open the jar—particularly if that smell is strong or "off"—you've kept it too long. Toss it and make a new batch.

GLOW TIPS

From Perfectly Pampered Celebrity Moms:

To pamper her body, mind, and spirit, super-plus model and fashion designer **Emme** says she scooped L'Occitane Shea Butter into an essential oil diffuser with almond and avocado oils, lit candles, and took a shower. "I exfoliate and deep-condition my hair, then get out of the shower and smooth on warm shea butter . . . everywhere!"

For overall body pampering, actress **Tisha Campbell-Martin** says that an all-natural body care line called Carol's Daughter was her favorite indulgence—and one, she says, that helped prevent stretch marks. "Their cocoa butter is rich and the oils are lightly scented and it's inexpensive—another good thing!" she says.

Award-winning beauty **Cate Blanchett** is a fan of skin care products by Dr. Hauschka, a line based on herbs, plants, and flowers. During pregnancy she pampered herself with his Rose Day Cream and Fitness Leg Spray, made of horse chestnut.

Itches, Bumps, and Rashes: What to Expect During Pregnancy

Among the more uncomfortable conditions associated with pregnancy are a number of skin rashes related to the hormonal and other physiologic changes that swing into action just after you conceive. While most of these problems are not dangerous, symptoms *can* range from mildly annoying to downright irritating. Some might even require medical attention. In a few rare instances they may even be confused with more serious problems that can have some potentially dangerous complications. For all these reasons, it's a good idea to familiarize yourself with the signs and symptoms and the self-care treatments that are safe to try.

To help you do just that, you can use the following guide. Prepared with medical data published by two of the world's top dermatologists— Dr. Chee Lok Goh, from the University of Singapore and the National Skin Center of Singapore, and Dr. Joseph C. Pierson, Chief of Dermatology, U.S. Military Academy—it can help you to better understand and pamper your pregnant body should any of these problems arise. Since skin problems often mimic each other, remember that it's always important to bring whatever symptoms you are experiencing to the attention of your doctor and get his or her advice on the best treatment options for you.

GLOW TIP

Itchy All Over

If your skin becomes dry and itchy all over, cut down on your shower time and use lukewarm water instead of hot. Switching from soap to moisturizing body wash can also help. Apply après-bath moisturizer while skin is still wet.

Nia Terezakis, M.D.

CONDITION #1: PRURIGO OF PREGNANCY (PP)

Often confused with heat rash or even sunburn, prurigo consists of tiny (1 to 2 millimeters) raised dots that are usually extremely itchy. One of the most common of pregnancy rashes—it occurs in 1 of every 300 pregnancies—it usually develops during the middle months and then disappears. In some women, however, it doesn't show up until the last few weeks of the third trimester, and lasts up to three weeks after childbirth. In the earlier form, the rash often appears on the upper half of your body, affecting your trunk, thighs, and upper arms but rarely your abdomen or buttocks. In the later form, the rash begins almost exclusively on your stomach, usually in the area where your stretch marks have occurred. After delivery, however, it can spread to the rest of your body and last for several weeks.

Although no one is certain what causes this rash, or why some women get it and others do not, doctors do know that it is generally not associated with any complications, either for you or your baby. But this doesn't mean that the itch might not be more than a little annoying. If it is, simple over-the-counter remedies may offer you the best relief. Check with your doctor about the use of aloe vera gel with a hint of mint, calamine lotion, or, if the itch is very intense, an over-the-counter hydrocortisone or antihistamine cream. While there is no evidence that perfumed creams or lotions are linked to this rash, doctors say that if you are experiencing any skin irritations during pregnancy, avoid all topical products containing heavy fragrance.

For all-natural itch relief, dip a washcloth in cold milk and apply to your skin for about five minutes. Milk has anti-inflammatory properties that can stop the vicious itch/scratch cycle. You can also try soaking in a warm (but not hot) bath to which you have added up to ½ cup of baking soda. Or try making a paste of baking soda and water and apply where skin feels the itchiest.

CONDITION #2: PUPPS (PRURITIC URTICARIA PAPULES AND PLAQUES OF PREGNANCY)

Affecting 1 in every 120 to 240 pregnant women is a condition known as pruritic urticaria papules and plaques of pregnancy (in Europe it's called polymorphic eruption of pregnancy). You, however, may know it by its more common name: PUPPS.

Usually developing in the latter half of pregnancy, often in the third trimester, PUPPS can cause a series of extremely itchy red bumps resembling hives—some of which can grow together into large plaques. Often the rash begins around the navel and follows the path of stretch marks, if you have them. Eventually it can spread to your thighs and sometimes your breasts, buttocks, even your arms. Your face, however, should not be affected.

No one is certain why PUPPS occurs, but if this is your first pregnancy, you are at greatest risk. However, don't rule it out just because you have given birth before. Studies show that up to 20 percent of women who develop PUPPS get it for the first time in a second or third pregnancy.

And while black women are seldom affected, if you are pregnant with twins or triplets you are at increased risk. Since at least some doctors believe that skin stretching may be at the root of PUPPS, it's not hard to see why the bigger your belly grows, the greater your risk of this problem. One study even revealed how mothers who gain excessive weight during their pregnancy have an increased risk of PUPPS—another good reason to keep an eye on those extra pregnancy pounds. Curiously, another study found that women who give birth to boys are twice as likely to develop PUPPS as women who have girls—but this finding has never been duplicated. More recently, doctors have identified evidence of fetal DNA in the skin cells of mothers who have PUPPS, indicating that some cells that cross the placenta from baby to mom could play a role in the rash.

Because there are no blood or urine tests to confirm PUPPS, it's important that your doctor perform a hands-on diagnosis. This is particularly important, since sometimes a PUPPS rash can resemble an allergic reaction to drugs or even food. On occasion, symptoms can mimic those of other, more serious skin diseases that can occur during pregnancy, so it's important that you do get a diagnosis soon after the rash appears.

PUPPS BODY CARE

While PUPPS may feel just awful, you can relax knowing that it's not serious: It won't harm you or baby, and it will likely disappear immediately after giving birth, sometimes within hours. Although doctors generally don't prescribe treatments for PUPPS, suggesting instead that you use either cold compresses to control itching or natural anti-itch remedies such as aloe vera gel, for some women medical treatment does become necessary. When this is the case, doctors normally prescribe a topical corticosteroid cream. If symptoms occur very late in your pregnancy and are somewhat overwhelming, your doctor may also prescribe an oral steroid medication or sometimes an antihistamine. In case you're wondering, analgesics like acetaminophen or aspirin won't help PUPPS.

What you can try on your own: calamine lotion, Caladryl (active ingredients: calamine, pramoxine HcL), Solarcaine (active ingredient: benzocaine), Solarcaine Aloe (active ingredient: lidocaine), Benadryl (active ingredient: diphenhydramine hydrochloride), Aveeno Anti-Itch Concentrated Lotion (active ingredients: calamine and camphor), Sarna Anti-Itch Lotion or Respite (active ingredients: camphor and menthol). Since these products obviously contain chemicals, make certain to **check with your doctor before using them**. To further reduce the irritation caused by PUPPS or any pregnancy rash, stay out of the direct path of an electric fan, even if it's the dead of summer and you're sweltering. Because the flow of air stimulates nerve endings, your itching is bound to escalate. Air-conditioning, on the other hand, provides a more even cooling effect that can alleviate discomfort. If you must use a fan, direct the air flow above or around you instead of directly on your body.

CONDITION #3: HERPES GESTATIONIS (HG)

Although its name may suggest otherwise, this skin condition is not related to any form of the herpes virus. It does, however, strongly resemble a herpes breakout, with sore, inflamed, fluid-filled blisters and lesions beginning around the navel and spreading out to other parts of the body.

An Expert's Opinion on

PREGNANCY RASH AND
BIRTH CONTROL PILLS

If you find that your herpes gestationis (HG) rash recurs after pregnancy—even years after you deliver—don't be too surprised, particularly if you are using birth control pills. According to Chicago dermatologist Dr. M. Joyce Rico, although symptoms of HG tend to regress spontaneously within days after delivery, the persistence of disease activity can continue deep within the body for years. As Dr. Rico explains, while you won't see or feel the rash, the antibodies that resulted from your first breakout remain in your system, waiting to be triggered into action. For some, she says, that trigger is oral contraceptives. To make certain that an HG recurrence is truly the source of your symptoms, never self-diagnose—see your doctor and get that biopsy. Since you are no longer pregnant, oral or topical steroids should heal you quickly. Then talk to your gynecologist about a different form of birth control.

Known in Europe as pemphigoid gestationis, HG is thought to be the result of an autoimmune disorder that develops when the skin makes antibodies against itself. Besides occurring during pregnancy, thyroid disorders, along with anemia (low red blood cell count), can increase the risks.

Most often HG breakouts begin on your navel, but they can quickly spread to other parts of your body. Although symptoms normally develop during pregnancy, studies show up to 25 percent of women develop this rash after delivery. Symptoms can also worsen just before or just after giving birth—but don't worry, it's not contagious, so your baby is not at risk. When HG is present during pregnancy, however, it can increase *your* risk of premature birth and, in rare instances, even endanger your baby's life by causing a number of pregnancy complications.

Because the symptoms of HG can be confused with those of chicken pox, shingles, dermatitis, or even a food or drug reaction, it is necessary to have a skin biopsy to confirm the diagnosis. Once diagnosed, symptoms can often be easily controlled with a topical steroid medication to reduce inflammation and topical antibiotics to control the threat of skin infection. Normally the lesions are confined to limited areas of the body, so you probably won't need to use an extensive amount of medication during treatment. And usually remission occurs spontaneously shortly after birth. However, if lesions are extensive either during pregnancy or right after, talk to your doctor about the use of oral prednisone, a steroid medication that can help control the breakouts internally.

WHEN A PREGNANCY RASH MEANS SOMETHING MORE

Occasionally itching skin can be a sign of systemic disease—a problem that exists somewhere inside your body. During pregnancy, it can be the result of a liver-related disorder known as intrahepatic cholestasis. In this instance, ducts that normally drain a fluid known as bile from your liver become blocked or swollen. As a result, liver inflammation develops.

While cholestasis can occur anytime after your twelfth week of pregnancy, it typically develops during the third trimester. The first sign is usually generalized body itching, including arms, legs, palms of your hands, soles of your feet, and even your scalp. Often you will feel worse at night and in the very early morning. Sometimes you may also develop a yellowy complexion color known as jaundice, which can appear about three weeks or more after the itching begins.

Although these symptoms may sound frightening, this condition is generally not dangerous for you. However, some studies have indicated an increased risk of premature birth and possibly some fetal distress in babies of mothers who developed cholestasis. Other studies, however, have shown no related problems.

To help diagnose this condition, your doctor can administer two liver enzyme tests: one measures levels of a compound known as bilirubin, the other measures bile acid. If cholestasis is diagnosed, your doctor may prescribe a medication known as cholestyramine to control itching. Normally the problem disappears spontaneously right after birth.

ITCHING AND NO RASH: WHAT TO DO

As disconcerting as a pregnancy rash is, what can be even more frustrating is an all-over body itch and no rash. Because there are no outward signs of inflammation, many women become fearful that their itching is all psychological and are too embarrassed to even talk to their doctor about it.

In reality, however, if you find yourself with itchy skin and nothing else, you may have a problem known as *pruritus gravidarum,* the "itch of pregnancy." Normally developing sometime in the third trimester, about 20 percent of pregnant women experience the curious phenomenon of the itch without the rash. Just because you have no little red bumps to show for your misery doesn't lessen the fact that you are most likely feeling very uncomfortable. While no one is certain what causes the problem, many dermatologists point to extremely stretched skin, which can also be dry and itchy. Obstetricians lean more toward hormonal activity as the cause, which they believe affects nerve endings in the skin that trigger the itch. Either way, both groups say that scratching is only going to make things worse; it won't stop your itch, and it could cause you to develop a nasty secondary skin infection.

While traditional antihistamines don't appear to offer much help, many women find relief with topical preparations designed to soothe the skin: applying a washcloth soaked in cool milk, taking a bath in honey and oatmeal, or simply slathering the skin with cocoa butter. You can also try products specifically formulated for pregnancy itches, including Bella Mamma's Pregnant Belly Oil with Lavender or Belli Cosmetics All Day Moisture Body Lotion. Or choose any body moisturizer that doesn't contain a lot of chemicals or fragrance, such as Orjene Cosmetics Fragrance-Free Elastin products. Check drugstore shelves for Lubriderm Lotion or Eucerin Daily Skin Therapy Plus Intensive Repair Cream. You can also talk to your doctor about trying Eucerin Itch Relief Moisturizing Spray. While most often the itch will subside on its own, if a rash eventually does show up, bring it to the attention of your doctor. And, rash or not, don't be afraid or embarrassed to mention your itchy skin at your next prenatal visit. It's something that should be documented on your medical chart.

The Glow Philosophy: Some Final Words

For many of you, pregnancy *will* be a time when you look and feel your very best. But even if your first trimester starts off on the wrong beauty foot, chances are good that midway through, you'll hit your stride and that glow *will* appear. If, however, for any reason things don't go quite as planned, remember that a little extra pampering at this time can go a long way in helping you to look and feel your best.

Even if you've never splurged on skin care or makeup products before, if you can, now may be the time to spend a little extra on yourself— and treat yourself to some of the luxuries you may have skipped over in the past. You may be surprised to discover just how good a little pampering can make you feel. Most important, when you feel good, your pregnancy and your baby will thrive.

You've Got Style

How to Be a Hot Mamma!

If you are like many women, from almost the moment you discovered the great news, your mind didn't stop spinning: Will my baby be healthy? What will he look like? Will she have my nose? What are we going to name him? Where will she sleep? And oh my gosh, I've got to stop drinking coffee this instant! As you probably have already figured out, there is seemingly no end to the number of thoughts—and questions—that will race through your head as the days unfold.

But as the news begins to sink in, and "I'M PREGNANT" slowly evolves into a much more quiet "I'm pregnant," still one more question is going to pop into your head: What the heck am I going to wear? And it's a question that can take on even more importance if you plan to work outside the home during your pregnancy and especially if your job requires that you keep to a specific dress code.

While finding the answer may not be quite as urgent as dealing with those issues that directly involve your health or even your comfort level, don't be quick to dismiss this important part of your pregnancy. As women, how we feel about ourselves, the image we project, even our confidence level is often intimately linked to how we look. The way we dress not only shows the world where we like to shop—it tells a little something about who we are and how we see ourselves. In terms of your career, your clothes help project your professional image, and in many instances are more intimately tied to how you act and react on the job than you might realize.

In the past, most women had to all but give up any sense of personal style soon after conception occurred. As white Peter Pan collars, pink and blue bows, and polka dots galore seemed to dominate the maternity fashion scene, there was little in the way of free choice. Thankfully, this is no longer the case. Today the world of maternity style is exploding with options—and enough choices to allow even the most fashion-conscious among us to find the clothes that suit our needs.

But as plentiful as these options can be, *finding* your special look can be a bit tricky. Not only will you have to choose clothing to suit your lifestyle and your budget, you're also going to have to build your new look around your changing body. Beginning with your breasts and heading straight for your tummy, it's clear that everything about you is going to grow: wider, thicker, and, yes, fatter. Nature, it seems, has a plan for you, and, in the end, nature is going to win! And sometimes that's going to mean making some serious changes in how you view the types of clothing that suit you best.

At the same time, however, accepting your new shape and size *doesn't* have to mean abandoning your sense of self or, just as important, your sense of style. What's that, you say, you didn't know you had a sense of style? Oh, but you do. Everything about the colors you choose, the fabrics you like to wear, the height of your heels and slouchiness or curves of your sweaters—these are all style elements that define who you are. And they are the same elements of style that can help you define the way you look during your pregnancy—as you continue to tell the world a little more about who you are!

Finding Your Pregnancy Style:
Where to Begin

Believe it or not, the best place to begin assembling your "new" look is right in your own clothes closet. It starts with giving your current wardrobe the once-over, while keeping your pregnant body in mind. Doing this will not only help you see the bigger picture of the kinds of clothes you like to wear (sporty outfits, conservative tailored looks, or a blend of eclectic chic), it will also help you to pull out those pieces that may do double duty by working during at least the first half of your pregnancy. Pay attention to any loose-fitting sweaters, blazers, T-shirts as well pants or skirts with any degree of stretch or elastic in the waist or fabric. Remember, spandex is your friend—and it may help your current wardrobe to serve you well into your second trimester.

Next up is to see how far your accessories will take you. Forget belts; they're not going to fit comfortably much past the first eight or ten weeks. But items such as scarves, shawls, hats, bags, socks, and especially jewelry not only turn even the simplest pregnancy basics into snazzy, stylish looks, they can also help you to carry on your prepregnancy sense of personal style. One dear friend pulled herself through an especially difficult pregnancy by wearing as many of her prepregnancy accessories as possible. She said it kept her in touch with who she was before she got pregnant, as it helped her to visualize that there *was* an end to the seemingly unending weight gain, fatigue, and bloating that came with carrying triplets.

Once you know what you have in terms of both clothing and accessories, it's time to do a little shopping. And if you're smart, you won't limit yourself to just one maternity store. Some of these shops—such as Pea in the Pod, Mimi Maternity, Baby Style, and Motherhood—carry such a wide variety of styles you could certainly find everything you need under one roof. But if you're not the type who would ordinarily buy your entire wardrobe at one store—even if it is Bloomingdale's or Saks—then I urge you not to confine yourself to one source for your maternity wear either.

In addition, realize that in many instances you can shop in non-maternity stores as well, by simply going up a few sizes. As long as the styles are not ultra–form-fitting or super tailored (lots of darts and seams aren't going to be so comfortable), you may find that the exact same type of outfits you wore before pregnancy still work for you now—only a few sizes larger. At the same time, don't go for the potato-sack look common in especially large clothes. They will only serve to make you look bigger.

Also, don't be quick to bypass chain stores or outlets, which can be terrific sources for great bargains on your maternity wear. The Gap, Old Navy, and even QVC now offer some great maternity garb that won't break your bank account. As long as you stick to basics—tops, skirts, and slacks in solid colors—you can mix and match with a few more expensive items, then use your own accessories to upgrade the whole look.

In all instances, however, the key is to choose items that resemble things you might normally have chosen when you weren't pregnant—the designs, fabrics, and colors should appeal to your personal sense of style. Above all, your new wardrobe shouldn't make you feel like you got dressed in the dark in someone else's closet.

You—from the Inside Out: Shopping for Pregnancy Lingerie

Regardless of how much or how little you spend on your pregnancy wardrobe, the one area where you probably shouldn't skimp is in your undergarments. While clearly, some stores go overboard in what they try to convince you that you need (will you really be all that comfortable in a pregnancy thong?), there are some basic undergarments that *can* make an important difference in not only how you look, but how you feel.

Among the most important is a well-made pregnancy bra. Depending on how quickly your breasts enlarge, you may have to change sizes or even styles more than once during your pregnancy, so it's not necessary to buy a lingerie wardrobe right from the start. That said, it's probably a good idea to do a little window-shopping early on in your pregnancy to become familiar with what's available. When the time comes for a new size or style, you'll have an idea where to go to find what you like and need.

For most women, a bra with wide-set straps that are also thicker in width helps give much-needed support while minimizing pressure on your shoulders. Remember that together, your breasts can gain as much as five pounds during pregnancy, which, in case you don't already know, can feel a lot like hanging a watermelon around your neck and expecting your shoulders to carry the weight! So, the thicker the straps, the more the extra weight will be distributed, which means the less your shoulders and upper back will feel the strain.

You should also seek out the smoothest, softest fabrics possible, choosing bras with a minimum of seaming in the cup area. In fact, the smoother and softer the cup is, the more comfortable your growing and tender breasts will feel. Also remember that you are going to need more coverage than you did before, to help support painful and tender breasts, so bypass the décolletage styles and instead look for a full cup style.

Also look for fabrics and styles that will hold up to repeated washing. Remember, you probably won't purchase as many pieces as you normally might have in your lingerie drawer, so each one you do buy is going to get more than the average number of washings. Styles with lots of lace or other trims, or thin or fragile fabrics, may not hold up as long as you need them. What can also help: Hand wash and line dry your pregnancy lingerie. Doing so puts less wear and tear on fabrics than a washer and dryer, the heat of which can also quickly beat down elastic and spandex.

BOTTOMS UP!

Whether you need to purchase pregnancy panties, or simply buy a larger version of what you already wear, is strictly a matter of personal taste. In fact, if you want to still wear those old bikinis and they feel comfortable, then feel free to do so—being pregnant doesn't have to mean starting every day by pulling on a pair of billowy Grandma Bloomers.

If you do purchase new panties, you may want to pay a little more attention to the fabrics, again looking for those that may hold up a little better with repeated washing. Also remember that you are likely to have extra vaginal discharge as your pregnancy progresses, as well as some degree of incontinence, so you'll want to choose fabrics that are easy to wash, dry quickly, and don't stain easily. You may also need to choose a style with substantial crotch width. If you want to wear a sanitary or incontinence pad during your pregnancy, it helps if the crotch is wide enough for the pad to fit comfortably and adhere.

The one speciality lingerie item you should definitely consider is maternity panty hose. It seems that no matter how large a size you choose in regular hose, the top is likely to slide off your belly and end up in an uncomfortable puddle at the top of your crotch. The hose may even tug down to the point where your stockings puddle around your ankles or at least bag significantly at your knees. Maternity panty hose have a wider, softer, stretchier top that can smooth up and over your tummy easily and remain relatively secure there for the whole day. Check the package for sizing information and make certain that what you buy is large enough to accommodate your tummy as well as your hips. What you don't want to do is load up on one size at the start of your pregnancy, since not only the size but the overall shape of your tummy will change.

Another must-have for many women: a pregnancy girdle. While you may have detested even the thought of wearing this type of garment before you conceived, you have to change your thinking now that baby is on the way. Not only will a pregnancy girdle help your clothes to look and fit better, the extra support it provides to your tummy and your back can help ease many pregnancy aches and pains and even prevent some from occurring at all.

But if you are tempted to skip the maternity department and instead shop for a regular girdle in a larger size, don't. While support is important, it's equally important that your stomach does not experience extreme compression. Most maternity girdles have ultra-stretchy, soft front panels that won't bind or cut your stomach, so they are both safer and more comfortable to wear.

There are several styles of maternity girdles to choose from, and what you select is often determined by your size and the degree of support you are seeking. For minimal uplift just under the tummy, choose a bikini or bikini-brief style. Either one tucks neatly underneath your stomach. The bikini brief can work through many more months of pregnancy, serving as an over-the-stomach girdle early on, then easily rolling down to a bikini in later months.

For greater back and stomach support—extremely important if you are carrying more than one baby or if you suffer from backaches—look for a "full" girdle, one designed to cover the entire front of your stomach up to the waist. Most usually have the added support of an elastic belt that runs across the upper back and down under the belly in the front.

This garment will help to both uplift and support your stomach, taking pressure off your back as well as your bladder.

Another slightly different version is frequently sold as a maternity back support. It's usually made of a heavier elastic material and has no panty. Instead, it wraps around the body, beginning at the lower back and moving to the front, where wide support straps wrap under the belly and close with a Velcro strip. Fully adjustable, it is another excellent way to give your stomach support while taking pressure off your lower back. Because it is adjustable, one of these can also pretty much last through your entire pregnancy.

You also may want to invest in a postpartum girdle for after your baby is born. These garments offer extra support under the stomach, while keeping waist compression to a minimum. Many also come with a snap closure on the crotch, allowing you to change a sanitary pad easily without having to pull the girdle down.

Pregnancy and Your Professional Style

For many women, the greatest pregnancy fashion challenge comes when choosing a work wardrobe. Depending on what you do and the confines of any corporate dress policies, finding the right clothes to suit your professional image can drive you to distraction. But it doesn't have to. With just a little forethought and some extra shopping time, you can quickly and easily pull together a stylish and polished look without spending a fortune. It begins by shopping with an open mind, while keeping some basic guidelines in mind.

1. *Stick to solid colors and similar fabrics to get away with fewer pieces.* If you also choose darker colors, you'll get more wear from each piece. Plus dark colors can help detract from your growing size. While nothing is going to hide that you are pregnant, you can keep from calling attention to yourself if you avoid loud prints, bright colors, and extremely tight clothes. You can change simple, basic pieces in black, navy, brown, camel, or gray by accenting them with scarves, jewelry, hats, and shoes in bright colors or prints.

2. *Avoid becoming a fashion tent.* While you may think that extra-large, full-cut tops and dresses will hide your size, they actually have the opposite effect. Remember, the larger the tent, the bigger the circus, so shop for clothing that is slim cut with some shape. The goal here is to develop a neat, pulled-together look that gently hugs your body without clinging. Also remember that any item with at least 5 percent Lycra (spandex) will not only fit better, but also be more comfortable to wear, and may even have more longevity. If you wear pants, choose styles with a slightly flared leg, which will help balance your figure. Skirts should be long enough to allow you to feel comfortable sitting in direct view of your boss. If you have great legs, don't be afraid to show them off with a slim-fitting knee-length skirt—just skip the minis and the slits up the side for now.

3. *Update your look with fashion jewelry.* Nothing says "this season" like a few well-chosen pieces of trendy fashion jewelry. Great earrings in colors that match your eyes will bring lots of attention to your face—and keep it away from your belly—while bracelets and necklaces will focus attention away from your outfit and onto your sense of style. And if pregnancy is keeping you from wearing this season's trendiest outfits, remember, for each new style there's a co-ordinating accessory, so going for half the look will help keep you looking up to date.

   Also important: You may want to start building a small collection of clip-on earrings, even if you have pierced ears. While it won't make much difference now, after baby is born, you'll love the idea of not having to worry about little fingers getting caught up in your pierced earrings and possibly tearing your ears.

4. *Never underestimate the power of a great jacket to give a polished, corporate edge to any pregnancy outfit.* You can start with any full-cut blazer you already own and it's perfectly okay to leave the bottom buttons open to make room for your growing belly. Later on, invest in one or two maternity jackets. Usually cut with a wider girth, in an unconstructed style, they will drape gracefully over your belly without making you look too large. Add a long scarf tied loosely

in the front, and no one will even notice what you're wearing underneath.

5. *Never underestimate the power of shoulder pads.* While the broad-shoulder power suits of the 1980s may be long gone, neat, well-balanced shoulders can do miraculous things for your figure, particularly during pregnancy. Look for pads that are medium in size with clean lines—either rounded or squared—in a dense foam that will hold its shape under any fabric, like Shape Essentials by Kathleen Kirkwood. They'll help your clothing fall more smoothly over your increasing bust size and give a neater, less rumpled and more professional look to your blouses and jackets.

6. *Choose clothing in substantial fabrics.* No matter what season you are pregnant, for a truly professional look, opt for garments made from fabrics with a substantial "hand," such as bouclé, twill, gabardine, or even cotton. Remember, substantial doesn't have to mean heavy, it just means finding items with more "body." A crisp, woven cotton shirt, for example, will look infinitely more professional than a flimsy knit top. In addition, the darker the color, the less likely little bumps and bulges will show through your clothes—including your belly button, which will also be growing larger and can protrude through some ultra-thin or ultra-soft fabrics.

7. *To complete your polished, professional look, opt for a shoe with at least a one-and-a-half-inch heel height.* Besides giving your look a more stylish edge, it's actually better for your back than flats.

Facing Another Pregnant Day

While it's true that there is a "glow" that comes with being pregnant, for more women than not, on more days than we'd like to think, looking our best takes a lot more than a quick pinch on the apples of our cheeks and a swipe of lip gloss.

At times pregnancy may present you with your *biggest* makeup challenges to date, with many of your old standby products absolutely refusing to give you even the slightest bit of help. Part of the reason has to do

An Expert's Opinion on

PREGNANCY ETIQUETTE

As you may have already noticed, there appears to be something about your being pregnant that sends other people's sensibilities flying. While a stranger or even an acquaintance would dare not rub his or her hand across your tummy and utter "Nice flat abs—lucky you!" that same person wouldn't think twice about patting your pregnant belly and making an inappropriate intimate comment.

At the same time, when it comes to acknowledging your pregnant status in places like a crowded bus or train, some folks can be amazingly shortsighted, ignoring your bulging belly and keeping the seat for themselves.

Much of the way in which you choose to deal with all these situations is part of your pregnancy style. To ensure that you do handle your state of grace with the utmost grace itself, *Good Housekeeping* magazine's etiquette doyenne Peggy Post (granddaughter of the late, great style maven Emily Post) says keep your sense of humor at all times—and tell people *nicely* when it's something you don't appreciate.

with some of the problems unique to pregnancy—such as a temporary change in your complexion type, carrying around a few excess gallons of water, or even a slight change in the shape of your face. All these things can make it suddenly more difficult to get the "look" you're used to seeing in the mirror.

The good news is that help is available, and there are things you can do to capitalize on your assets and get the glow going—or apply it, if necessary, in no time flat! To help get you thinking in the right direction, some of the world's best beauty experts, including celebrity makeup artists Laura Geller, Bobbi Brown, and Holly Stougard-Mordini, offer you their advice for solving some of the most frustrating pregnancy makeup dilemmas.

"I've been poked or prodded enough" and "I don't like my stomach touched, I'm sure you understand" are two phrases she says you may want to commit to memory. And don't be afraid to take the direct route to short-circuit a conversation if folks comment about any aspect of your pregnancy—particularly your shape, size, or even your appetite.

If you're feeling a little feisty, Post advises that you can reply: "I guess you've never had a child, or you'd realize just how happy—and hungry—I am!" Since, she says, most folks take their conversation cues from the mother, it's important that you politely let people know how you feel.

When it comes to common everyday courtesies, such as giving a pregnant woman a seat on the bus, Post says don't expect everyone to automatically yield to your needs, even if those needs are obvious.

For sitting strangers, Post says, it is thoughtful, though not mandatory, to offer to give a pregnant woman a seat. If no one makes the offer, she advises that you just pick out whoever looks as if she or he could tolerate standing best (don't ask a senior, for example), simply mention that you are pregnant, and ask if the person would mind giving up his or her seat. Failing that, wear comfortable shoes, open your coat, and sigh a lot.

Quick Fixes for Your Pregnant Face: The Six Most Common Problems and How to Solve Them

PROBLEM #1: PUFFY SWOLLEN EYES/DARK CIRCLES

- *Diffuse Under Eye Concealer and Lightener by Smashbox.* A double-ended wand that features a golden color treatment stick with antipuff, anti–dark circle properties on one end and a light, whipped-cream concealer on the other. Used together, they give you a treatment and a cosmetic in one quick swipe—and because it is a treatment, effects are cumulative. The more you use it, the better you look! In color numbers 2 (light), 4 (medium), and 6 (dark).

- *TV Touch Medium Light Concealer Cream and Multi Color Conceal Wheel by Laura Geller.* Cream products that won't cake or collect in fine lines, they can cover all but the darkest circles. The multicolor wheel lets you custom blend your shade, so as your complexion color changes through pregnancy, you won't have to buy a new product.

- *Maybelline True Illusion Undetectable Creme Concealer.* Perfect for light coverage that never looks cakey or dry. Available in light or medium, it has a natural yellow tone that helps combat dark circles and skin discoloration.

- *Max Factor Erace.* One of the first camouflage products on the market and, some say, still the best. The coverage is heavy—it can cover even a birth mark or a pregnancy mask—but if you apply a good moisturizer first, then finish with a light layer of translucent powder, the coverage says fresh and lasts all day. In three traditional shades: fair, natural, and medium.

EXTRA GLOW TIP

Pregnancy Glam

To make even the sleepiest, puffiest pregnancy eyes look wide awake and brighter, line the bottom rim with a soft, white eyeliner pencil.

For fuller lips, blend a touch of concealer or highlighter at the bow of your lips and right under the lower lip.

For long-lasting lipstick try Chapstick as a primer under color. The waxiness in Chapstick smooths the lip surface, fills in tiny lines, and will help hold color on your lips longer.

Peter Lamas, international celebrity makeup artist, founder BeautyWalk.com

PROBLEM #2: SKIN FATIGUE

Tired, dull-looking skin, with a sallow or green cast or ashy coloring.

- *Artificial Light by Smashbox Cosmetics.* Facial-fresh look without the time, expense, and hassle, this nearly colorless product will put on the glow no matter how you feel. Infused with good-for-your-skin ingredients like green tea and ginkgo biloba (a natural radiance booster), plus vitamins A and E, you can use it right out of the bottle on clean skin, or mix it with foundation for a glow that will make even the Mona Lisa jealous. Available in four shades: Diffuse (a pearlized noncolor for all complexions), Glow (a sheer bronze—perfect for African American and Hispanic skin tones), Glare (a sheer rosy pink that bathes your face in the most flattering light possible), and Reflect (for a sheer golden glow on light, medium, and dark complexions).

  One caveat: This product has a pleasant but very strong fragrance, so be certain to give it the sniff test before you buy, particularly if you are ultra sensitive to perfumes right now.

- *Skin Spackle by Laura Geller.* No matter how bad your complexion may look or feel, Spackle will even out skin tone even when heartburn and bathroom runs have kept you up all night. An oil-free skin primer that can be used alone or in conjunction with your favorite moisturizer, it can turn even the dullest, sleepiest pregnancy complexion into a smooth canvas that allows makeup to glide on and stay on. With Spackle, you can use less foundation and even less blush and still have a flawless complexion. Colorless—so one product is right for every skin color.

- *Revlon SkinLights Face Illuminator.* Available in seven shades from Bare Light (a dewy, angel-light glow) to Bronze Light (a deep golden shade perfect for women of color), you can apply this product instead of moisturizer or right along with it, or wear it with foundation or alone, for shimmering skin that's not sparkly but definitely glowing. To perk up an ashy or green cast complexion, try Peach Lights or Pink Lights.

※ **EXTRA GLOW TIP** 〜〜〜〜〜〜〜〜〜〜〜〜

An Eye for Looking Good

If your pregnant cheeks are starting to puff, don't mess with streaky contours and dark powders. Instead, divert attention to the eyes by framing the face with great brows. Add liner to your lids and highlighter above and below the brow bone, and no one will notice you have walnuts in your cheeks!

Holly Stougard-Mardini, Smashbox Cosmetics

〜〜〜〜〜〜〜〜〜〜〜〜〜〜〜〜〜〜〜〜〜

PROBLEM #3: NO GLOW

- *Skin Tint by Smashbox Cosmetics.* If you're looking to put on a glow without putting on a face full of color, look to Skin Tint for that just-came-in-from-a-walk-on-the-beach glow. It's a sheer gel stick that creates a healthy-looking flush of color that appears to come from within (you don't actually see any product on your face the way you would see a blush). To apply, smile (even if you don't feel like it), gel up the apples of your cheeks, and blend with your fingertips. And because it's oil-free, you can use it even on super oily pregnant skin. Colors include Infra Red (a sheer cherry); Ultra Violet (a sheer berry that looks very dark in the case but in fact comes out a gloriously natural rosy color); Heat (a coral watermelon—and Holly Stougard-Mordini's favorite for a light pregnancy glow); and Lit (a sheer bronze, perfect for Hispanic and African American skin).

- *Cream Blush Stick by Bobbi Brown.* What makes this product particularly unique is not only the complexion-friendly shades (they are formulated to be skin-tone correct) but also the creamy formulations that help them glide on evenly so color looks natural. Available in six shades; try Soft Pink, Sand Pink, or Pale Pink to perk up a sallow or pale complexion.

- *Burt's Bees Blushing Creme with Vitamin E.* This super-moisturized cream blush offers coverage along with color without a cakey, dry look. Perfect to combat a dry pregnancy complexion with color that goes on smooth and looks natural. Plus, the vitamin E is good for your skin. In four shades, including Courage (a clear pink), Enthusiasm (a soft rosy glow), Tenderness (a barely there peach), and Clarity (a just-kissed-by-the-sun peach).

- **Sephora Aqua Tints.** A water-based product that offers the sheerest whisper of color, you'll get a glow that will last all day without touch-ups. Because it's a liquid stain, it grabs onto skin and stays put. But because colors are sheer, you'll never get that Kewpie doll overblushed look. The colors look dark in the bottle but come out much lighter on your skin. Experiment first on the back of your hand to find the right application. Available in six clear, sheer colors, beauty editors are raving about Auburn, a hint of a sun-kissed look all year long.

PROBLEM #4: DRY, CRACKED LIPS

- **Vibran C Lip Treatment by Laura Geller.** Because you are actually taking more breaths during pregnancy—and your breathing is more shallow—lips can easily get dry and cracked. This is particularly true during labor—some women actually end up with cracked, bleeding lips after giving birth. One solution is this super-emollient vitamin C stick for the mouth—a colorless glaze of moisture that can keep lips from chapping, peeling, drying, and hurting, winter or summer. Hint: Pack one in your labor bag for delivery day—you'll thank me!

- **Emulsion Lip Exfoliant and Lip Therapy by Smashbox.** A revolutionary pair of lip products that exfoliate and then moisturize for a smooth, glossy, pouty look that really lasts. The exfoliating cream combines sugar with poppy seeds to gently scrub away dry, dead skin. To kick it up a notch, they add a mood-elevating, nausea-busting peppermint scent that, remarkably, lingers on your lips even after the treatment is done, and tastes fabulous. Finish with the Lip Treatment—a super-emollient stick that combines honey, shea butter, and an SPF of 15 to seal in softness *and* protection.

- *Blistex Complete Moisture Lip Balm or Blistex Lip Revitalizer.* Neither product will add any color to your lips, but they can heal faster and protect better than almost anything on the market, with ultra-fast results. The balm contains an SPF of 30 to protect lips from the sun. Great to wear over lipstick—or try putting on the Blistex first, add lipstick, blot, then finish with a second coat of Blistex for conditioning color that really lasts.

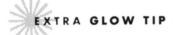

EXTRA GLOW TIP

Let Your Lips Do the Talking

To keep a natural lip line and still get that fully, pouty, sexy mouth, put lipstick on first, then go back and follow your natural lip line with a lip pencil in a color that is one or two shades deeper than your lipstick. Finish by adding more lipstick and then blending it all together, for a naturally full lip line without being obvious. If you don't have time to do anything else, line lips with a berry pencil and add a sheer bright berry, pink, or mauve lipstick for an instant complexion "pick-me-up."

Holly Stougard-Mordini, Smashbox Cosmetics

PROBLEM #5: OILY SKIN, FOUNDATION WON'T STAY PUT, BLUSH TURNS COLOR

- *Anti Shine by Smashbox.* There's no coverage here, but put Anti Shine on clean skin and watch the oil spills disappear—and stay away for hours! The revolution is in the drying effects, which, while soaking up the oil, *won't* pull out moisture. Plus, it leaves skin feeling cool and calm. The bottom line: Skin looks dewy fresh, without the greasies—which in turn can make foundations last longer and keep blush colors from turning. Available in three tints: Neutral (zero color), Light (with a pale beige tint), Medium (for Hispanic, Asian, and African American skin). For quick touch-ups during the day, try Photo Matte, a light, pressed powder with oil-blotting properties designed to minimize pores and keep the shine away.

- *Invisible Blotting Powder by Laura Geller.* Made from pure ground rice, this ultra-lightweight pressed powder works as a quick touch-up during the day or to set makeup in the morning. It absorbs excess oil, then disappears on your skin, so you don't have the traditional cakey, pasty look that powder can cause. One shade, translucent, works well on all skin types. Use alone, or in conjunction with Laura Geller Blotting Papers—thin sheets of pure rice paper that you press on skin to blot up the oil spills and take away the greasies.

- *Sephora Face Blotting Sheets.* Beauty-salon quality at a drugstore price, these dainty little wisps of tissue will keep even the oiliest complexions under control without streaking your foundation or wrecking your blush. They come in a handy purse dispenser for use anywhere and everywhere. Use alone or with Sephora's All Over Skins—a cornstarch-based pressed face powder that soaks up the greasies without leaving you looking like you fell in a vat of cake flour. Unlike other unishade translucents, this one comes in seven glorious colors from pale beige to deep tan, suitable for women of every complexion.

PROBLEM #6: ULTRA-DRY PARCHED SKIN THAT FLARES WITH EVEN A LITTLE MAKEUP

- *Extra Soothing Balm by Bobbi Brown.* Nothing counteracts that pregnancy glow more than dry, arid skin. But you can bring back your natural color and find the glow that's been hiding with products called "skin balms." And if you've never tried one, you won't believe the difference in your skin. A thick, highly dense, super-moisturizer infused with botanicals that can naturally add a radiant glow to your complexion, Extra Soothing Balm is like a cool glass of water for a hot, thirsty face. The best part: It can be applied right over your makeup midday for an instant pick-me-up.

- *Serious Skin Care Glucosamine Acid-Free Skin Products.* A collection of moisturizers, cleansers, scrubs, and even mini-peels designed for ultra-sensitive skin. If you can't or don't want to use an alpha hydroxy acid, the glucosamine products in this collection can accomplish much the same thing without disturbing ultra-sensitive pregnant skin.

- *Fresh Glow Creme Foundation by Bobbi Brown.* A lightweight, whipped foundation cream loaded with moisturizers and other good-for-your-skin ingredients, it keeps dry skin looking fresh and glowing without inflaming even the most stressed complexion. Available in eight skin-correct colors from ivory to deep espresso.

- *L'Oréal Feel Naturale Liquid Makeup.* This creamy formula not only offers a whisper of color, but it soothes your skin with vitamin E, moisturizes like crazy, and utilizes light-refracting particles for a prismlike quality that fools the eye by focusing away from all those imperfections. The end result is that skin glows and stays moist all day. In a variety of shades, from light beige to deep tan, it's suitable for all complexion colors.

GLOW TIP

Color Therapy

The moment you find out you're pregnant, go makeup shopping! Once your pregnancy is under way, you might discover that you need to perk up your complexion, and nothing does it better than a brighter color blush and lipstick.

Look for colors that are similar to what you normally use, in a shade or two lighter—or switch from peach tones to pink tones to take on a bit more of the rosy glow. Complement the look with equally bright lipstick—and look for products with texture, like a glossy finish, which gives off a youthful glow and lightens up your whole face.

Laura Geller, celebrity makeup artist, director, Laura Geller Cosmetics

Hair Today, Gone Tomorrow

Perhaps nothing screams "personal style" more than a great haircut. In fact, how you wear your hair—including not only the cut, but the color and even the overall style—is a great way to express your individuality and say a little something about who you are. And for many women, pregnancy turns out to be one never-ending really great hair day. As estrogen levels soar, a complex network of biochemical changes kick into high gear, almost overnight, so hair is thicker, shinier, and infinitely easier to manage.

Others are not so lucky. Pregnancy hormones can also wreak havoc with hair, tossing your personal style right out the window. Your first trimester can find you battling a severe case of the "greasies," as hair suddenly gets oilier than ever before. As your pregnancy progresses, straight or curly hair may go dry and frizzy, particularly late in the second or early in the third trimester. Hair that is already dry before pregnancy can become so brittle, you can even experience some breakage.

And while many women welcome the extra body that comes from having more hair during pregnancy—hormones again, sending a signal that stops the normal shedding process—those with already thick or heavy manes may find the extra strands add so much weight and bulk that their favorite cut no longer looks right and styling becomes almost impossible.

For still others, hair problems that existed before pregnancy are magnified after conception. Oily hair gets oilier, dry hair gets drier, hair that was hard to manage before can take on a whole new and unruly life of its own. Any or all of these problems may be further complicated by a hesitancy on your part to use some of the chemical hair products and treatments you previously relied on—items such as dyes or perms or even some styling aids.

So, what's a pregnant girl to do? With just a few changes to your hair care routine and perhaps a few new or different products, you can not only avoid many problems, but also pick up a few style tricks and tips that will serve you well after baby is born.

Solving Your Pregnancy Hair Problems: Where to Begin

Although it can seem like a painfully obvious idea, whether you are pregnant or not, the most basic of all your hair care regimens starts with choosing the correct shampoo. As elementary as this sounds, hairdressers around the globe say the majority of women simply don't use the right kind of products—one reason we can have so much trouble styling our own hair, particularly during pregnancy. So what should you look for? First and foremost, think gentle. While pregnancy hormones, particularly during the first trimester, may cause your hair to seem greasier and even dirtier than usual, unless you work in a coal mine, gentle, daily cleansing with a mild product is all you'll ever really need regardless of your hair type.

According to hair researcher Dr. Kevin J. McElwee, the kindest, gentlest shampoos must include at least some of the following ingredients, which should be listed on the product label:

sorbitol esters

polyglycerol ether

betaines

alkyl imidazoline

alkyl-amino acids

anything with the word "tween" in the name (tween-20, tween-80)

Trichologist Phillip Kingsley advises looking for shampoos that replace harsh detergent-like ingredients such as sodium lauryl sulfate and sodium laureth sulfate with kinder, gentler ingredients such as triehanolamine lauryl sulfate. This is good advice whether you are pregnant or not, but again, it may have the most value during your first trimester, when your hair, like your body, is getting "used to" hormonal changes.

You should also try to avoid products containing flash foamers—chemicals that do nothing except make your shampoo create more foam—which, by the way, won't get your hair any cleaner. Flash foaming and other harsh chemicals you may want to avoid include:

All terms with chemical suffixes ending in DEA or MEA (cocamide DEA or MEA, lauramide DEA or LEA or soyamide DEA)

cocamidopropyl betaine and cocamide MEA

cocamidopropylamine oxide

lauramine oxide

Since one trip down the shampoo aisle of your drugstore will tell you it's almost impossible to avoid all these chemicals completely, the next best thing is to limit as many as you can. Also look for products where the most questionable chemicals are as far down on the ingredient list as possible, meaning there is less in the product.

Now, if you're starting to think that maybe baby shampoo might just be the ticket for a mother-to-be, think again. If your hair isn't very dirty or very oily, it might work. However, these products are best suited for very low oil production and hair that doesn't get very dirty—both of which are true for babies, but not usually for Mom. Most hairdressers agree that for women with normal oil production, baby shampoo won't do the job. So skip it and instead opt for a gentle adult shampoo, such as those slated for dry or color-treated hair.

To get the best overall cleansing, particularly if you use a lot of styling aids, a clarifying shampoo can be your best choice—but don't use it every time you wash your hair. Although it can temporarily boost volume—mostly by removing traces of residue that weigh hair down—used too often it can cause some real damage, as the shampoo strips the protective oil barrier off each strand of hair.

A safer way to remove hair buildup and increase body: Add a handful of baking soda to your regular shampoo. This will help "lift" all the styling product from your hair without damaging your hair shaft, and turn any wash into a clarifying treatment.

GLOW TIP

Don't Overdo It

Don't shampoo your hair every day. Natural oils can condition your scalp and your hair naturally. If you do use a conditioner, use it only where your hair needs it. If you have thin and/or limp hair, condition the ends of your hair only. This way the conditioner won't weigh your hair down.

Robert Stuart Salon, New York City

Taming the Tiger in Your Hair: What Can Help

If pregnancy has left your hair frizzy, dry, difficult to style, or hard to curl, you may be in need of a hair moisturizer. Not to be confused with oil, moisture is what keeps hair supple and soft—taming and controlling the outside layer or "cuticle" of each strand and allowing it to lie flat and smooth.

According to Dr. John Gray, director of the Oxford Hair Foundation, look for products containing collagen or derived from silk amino acids, pathenol, or other derivatives of vitamin B_5. Any of these can easily penetrate hair strands and dramatically increase moisture content. Often sold as hair "masks," they go on like a traditional facial mask and remain on the hair for anywhere from five to twenty minutes.

If pregnancy has left your hair looking and feeling limp and fine, look for conditioners and moisturizers in a gel or clear liquid form rather than a paste or opaque creme. Ideally, they will be less weighty so they won't bog hair down, but still offer protection from the elements. If you permed, relaxed, or colored your hair just before getting pregnant, conditioners containing some form of hydrolyzed protein (check the ingredient label) can increase the strength of your hair shaft by up to 5 percent. This, in turn, may help decrease your risk of breakage until new hair starts to grow in. In fact, the more damaged your hair is, the easier it will be for the proteins to penetrate the outside layer and get inside, where they can

An Expert's Opinion on

DRASTIC HAIR CHANGES AND PREGNANCY

Looking for a new "do" to take you through pregnancy? Don't think drastic change, says renowned hair care expert George Michael, who also advises keeping long hair long. And if your hair is short at the start of your pregnancy, he says, let it grow. The reason, says Michael, is that long hair needs less maintenance—something you are going to definitely appreciate once your baby is born. For example, long hair doesn't have to be washed as frequently, since brushing distributes natural oils through each strand, helping to keep it from building up on the scalp. With short hair, however, oil doesn't have far to travel before it reaches the tips, so it's more likely to build up and look and feel greasier and ultimately be harder to manage. In addition, while pregnancy hormones can make hair seem thicker, because shedding stops, hair growth also slows down. If you do clip your locks during pregnancy, expect that it will take longer to grow back.

do the most good. This fact may be especially important to remember during your postpartum recovery, when hormonal shifts will cause you to lose the extra hairs you gained during pregnancy. At that time you'll want to do all you can to encourage healthy new hair growth.

Caring for Your Pregnant Hair Naturally

While it's likely you may already have a personal stash of favorite hair care goodies, if you are like many women, once pregnant you may find yourself gravitating toward more nature-based products. In an effort to avoid chemicals that could, at least theoretically, interfere with your pregnancy on some level, you may want to treat your hair to the best of what Mother Nature has to offer. While you can find many nature-based products in health food stores or even some on drugstore shelves, there are a number of natural hair care recipes you can whip up right in your own kitchen.

EXTRA GLOW TIP

Hair Loss vs. Hair Breakage

There is a distinct difference between hair loss and hair breakage. Learning to tell the two apart can save you much anxiety during pregnancy and during your postpartum period, when hair loss may become a real issue. Here's how to tell the difference:

Hair breakage is when the hair fractures on the ends or at any point throughout the length of the hair strand. Split ends are among the most common cause. The only cure for split ends is to cut them off.

Hair loss is when the hair comes out completely from the root of the follicle. Conditioning, treatment, and cutting off portions of damaged hair are among the most beneficial alternatives to restoring damaged hair.

House of Hair, Brooklyn, New York

GLOW TIP

Protecting Your Pregnant Hair

Never wrap hair in a towel turban when you get out of the shower. The added friction can knot and damage vulnerable wet hair. Instead, carefully blot hair dry.

A good thing to try: Once or twice a week, rub conditioner into dry hair *before* washing. This will allow the product time to penetrate the strands of hair before the water dilutes it, adding a little extra conditioning. After shampooing, rub in a leave-in conditioner on the ends of your hair. Always blow-dry with the air flow going down the hair (away from face) to get the shiniest and most manageable results.

The Hair Studio, Berkeley Springs, West Virginia

To help get you started, here are a variety of tips and recipes for everything from conditioners to styling aids.

NATURAL STYLING AIDS

ALL-NATURAL CONDITIONER

From Beverly Hills hair guru Tina Cassaday: Combine in a blender:

2 ounces of purified (or bottled) water

½ banana (a potassium-rich source of moisture)

1 tablespoon of plain yogurt (for calcium)

1 drop to 1 teaspoon of honey (for trace minerals)

¼ cantaloupe (for vitamins C and A)

1 tablespoon sweetened condensed milk (for vitamins A and D)

1 teaspoon of wheat germ oil (for thiamin and more)

Blend on medium for ten seconds; apply to hair in a downward motion and leave on for forty-five minutes, or longer if your hair is very dry or broken. Rinse off with warm water, then shampoo and rinse again with cool water to seal in hair cuticles.

BEAT THE FRIZZIES AND GAIN VOLUME

- For extra zip to zap those frizzies, try adding ¼ cup of honey and 1 tablespoon of almond oil to ½ cup of your favorite conditioner. Mix the ingredients well, pour on damp hair, let set for twenty minutes, then rinse thoroughly.

- To give your pregnant hair instant volume, try parting it to the right. Experts say most hair follicles grow from left to right, so a right part pushes hair against the natural angle of growth, adding instant height and body. A middle part puts additional stress on hair where it's the weakest and also accentuates any irregularities in facial structure.

- To naturally increase hair's body, add 1 cup of flat beer to 3 cups of water. Pour on hair, let set five minutes, then thoroughly rinse. The beer's protein and yeast content will make hair appear thicker and fuller.

- To reduce oiliness and boost fine limp hair, mix 1 teaspoon of lemon or lime juice into ½ cup of water. Spritz onto hair, massage into scalp, let sit for up to twenty minutes, and rinse thoroughly.

CITRUS HAIR SPRAY

Chop 1 lemon (for normal to oily hair) or 1 orange (for dry hair) and place in a pot with 2 cups of cold water. Bring to a boil and continue cooking until about 1 cup of water remains (about half the original amount). Remove from heat and cool, strain through fine cheesecloth, and pour into a pump spray bottle. Store in the refrigerator. If the spray is too sticky, dilute it with water. You can also add 1 ounce of rubbing alcohol as a preservative to keep up to 2 weeks unrefrigerated. Use in place of regular or even superhold store-bought hair spray.

NATURAL MOUSSE/GEL

Dissolve ½ to 1 teaspoon of unflavored gelatin in 1 cup of boiling water. Let sit at room temperature until it begins to thicken. Rub onto wet or dry hair and blow dry as usual.

NATURAL DANDRUFF CONTROL

For an all-natural dandruff treatment, herbal experts advise a rinse of ½ cup of water mixed with ½ cup of white vinegar. Apply directly to scalp prior to shampooing and let set about five minutes. Shampoo as usual. Apply treatment twice weekly.

GLOW TIP

Extra-high-impact volume can be yours without chemicals if you simply shampoo or at least rinse your hair with cold water. It pulls shampoo off each strand, making hair cleaner and automatically adding more body. For instant volume, no matter your hair type or texture, towel dry first, then apply blow-dry lotion at the roots only. Flip head forward, and blow dry from the bottom up. Flip head back and smooth the ends with a brush.

Sex in the City stylists Wayne Herdon and Mandy Lyons

Tuning Out the Static

If you brush your hair and it pretty near stands on end, then there's a good chance you're plagued with static electricity, a problem that can become quite common in the third trimester. The reason is that, as your pregnancy progresses, so does your baby's need for water. If you're not consuming enough liquid, your baby will pull that water from your skin and hair, leaving both drier than usual. When hair is dry, it sets the stage for static electricity to occur. Problems can multiply if you are pregnant in the winter months, when colder temperatures and hot air heat seem to conspire to dry out hair and skin and make static worse.

What can help: spraying your brush with a leave-on conditioner or hair spray before you style. You can also try a brush with natural bristles and a wooden handle, which helps reduce the formation of static during brushing. And, if you set your hair dryer on cool for the last third of your drying time, or rinse your hair in cool water when you conclude shampooing, you can control frizzies as well as static. Or try a final rinse that combines two tablespoons of vinegar with two cups of water. The extra acid in the vinegar will help cut the static once hair is dry.

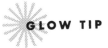

GLOW TIP

Better than a Swimcap!

Before swimming, always wet hair first with spring or tap water. The water acts as a barrier and reduces the amount of chlorine that hair absorbs from pool water.

Aristacutz Salon, Chelmsford, England

GLOW TIP

Make Long Hair Stronger

Brush hair only when it's dry. Hair is weakest when it is wet, and brushing can easily damage it. Even when hair is dry, always comb before brushing. To comb hair properly: Separate into small sections and, using a wide-tooth comb, work the hair from the ends down, in one direction only.

The Long Hair Group, New York City

Adding on Some Hair Style

If dealing with your pregnant hair becomes impossible—or you simply don't have the time to fuss—don't overlook the help you can get from synthetic hair add-ons. An entirely brand-new class of ultra-hip synthetic hair products, from braids to ponytails to classic chignons and buns, they can instantly turn a bad hair day into sheer joy.

Most of these pieces come complete with a heavy-duty "butterfly" clip that allows you to simply pull your hair back in an elastic band and instantly attach styled and luxurious full hair. If your own hair is ultra-short, slick the sides back using a gel, then clip the add-on to the hair at the crown. Some pieces—like the new Toni Twist (see Resource Center)—are an instant and sophisticated bun on an elastic band that attaches as quickly and easily as a traditional ribbon scrunchie. Plus, colors for both the Toni Twist and the Tony Tail (a two-for-one sleek and shag clip-on ponytail) are blended with sixteen different shades, so all you have to do is come close to your basic hair color and you've got an ideal match with natural-looking highlights that also perk up your complexion. If uber-matching is your thing, look for a wide selection of well-priced hair add-ons by Paula Young (see Resource Center). Most styles are available in up to twenty-five specific colors designed to match almost any hair color exactly.

Made of a natural-looking synthetic hair product, most of these pieces wash and dry in about an hour, and require no other maintenance. While they work fantastically during pregnancy, they turn into a *real life-saver* in the days and weeks following childbirth, when washing and styling your hair might be difficult. Another bonus: If you pack one of these hair add-ons in your labor bag, you'll have the absolute best look-ing "new mom–new baby" pictures on the block!

Dying for a Change:
Hair Color and Your Pregnancy

If you're like many women, bleaching, dying, or highlighting your hair may be a regular part of your beauty regime. And if you're like most preg-nant women, you probably have some hesitation or even fear about con-tinuing to color your hair while baby is in tow. Although research into the effects of hair coloring on baby's health is still somewhat limited, as recently as December 2001 the American College of Obstetricians and Gynecologists issued a statement indicating that hair dyes are most likely safe and that women needn't be afraid to color their world during preg-nancy. The New York Office of the Organization of Teratology Informa-tion Service concurs that coloring your hair probably is safe. Even the text *Occupational and Environmental Reproductive Hazards: A Guide for Clini-cians* does not list any hair dye as a known or suspected cause of birth de-fects.

Despite that, those in the maternity trenches—doctors, nurses, and midwives—often recommend that you approach hair coloring with caution during pregnancy. Because the dye is absorbed through the scalp and into the body (it can be identified in urine), many medical experts are hesitant to give carte blanche to hair coloring during all three trimesters.

The bottom line: Most physicians agree that if you hold off coloring your hair with permanent dyes during the first trimester—a time when your baby is undergoing important neurological developments—you can probably safely resume coloring in the second or third trimester. What's more, if you color your hair at home, choose products with the least number of chemicals and always work in a well-ventilated room, wearing gloves while handling the mixture. If you have your hair done in a salon, request the first appointment in the morning on the least busy day—when you are least likely to suffer excessive chemical exposure.

Hair Coloring Alternatives

If you don't want to take a chance on coloring your whole head of hair, you may want to consider adding highlights—a great way of accenting your color and bringing light to the face, not to mention a little pregnancy glow! Because highlighting, painting, or even frosting hair involves applying the chemicals one-half to one inch from your roots, they don't ever touch your scalp. So they can't get into your bloodstream. And since you won't see outgrowth as quickly, you can easily allow eight weeks or more between appointments—and that minimizes your salon exposures as well.

If you colored your hair before pregnancy but want to ease up on treatments until after baby is born, look for a semipermanent dye containing low or no ammonia and low or no peroxide. These products can help blend the different colors of your hair and make roots appear less obvious. What can also help: color-enhancing shampoos. Designed to deposit temporary color, they can significantly extend the time between hair colorings.

Finally, you can also try a hair mascara. A relatively new term for a product that's been around a while, these are tubes filled with temporary color that is applied with a thick mascara-like wand. Available in a variety of shades—including naturals like blonde, brunette, and redhead, and fun shades like purple, pink, gold, and silver—a quick swipe gives you a bold or shy streak that lasts until your next shampoo. Because they coat only the outside layer of your hair and don't get anywhere near your scalp, they are very safe to use. The wands are also faster, easier, and safer than spray-on temporary color—there are no fumes to inhale—so they can work great to touch up roots. Or you can try a hair coloring stick—a lipsticklike tube with concentrated temporary color you apply directly on your roots.

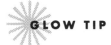

GLOW TIP

Easy Does It

Be extra gentle when brushing hair that is relaxed, color treated, or permed, since it's weaker from the chemical processing. When your hair color or a perm is growing out, it is weakest where the processed hair meets the new growth, and improper brushing may snap the strands at this point.

Jazma Hair Care, Ontario, Canada

Perming, Straightening, and Pregnancy

Much like coloring, perming or relaxing hair requires the use of products containing a plethora of chemicals—solutions strong enough to lift your hair cuticle, penetrate the hair shaft, and literally change the shape of your hair. All of the chemicals used in hair straightening or perming are applied to the scalp and can be absorbed into the bloodstream.

While there is little in the way of scientific information on the safety of perming or relaxing solutions while pregnant, perhaps the most convincing evidence against their use is that which comes directly from the beauty industry. Hairdressers caution that because pregnancy hormones frequently interfere with, or even change, the way your hair reacts to perming or relaxing solutions, you could easily end up with a look that is quite opposite of what you expected. Hair can get frizzy or straight instead of curly, or kinky and frizzy instead of straight.

Mother *Nature* Knows Best

NATURAL HAIR COLORING

If you are tempted by ads from health food stores or "all-natural" product lines to try what is often referred to as vegetable dyes, listen up: Hair color experts and medical experts alike caution "buyer beware." According to certified nurse midwife Ann Linden, in addition to herbs and other natural ingredients listed on the package, these products often contain many of the same synthetic chemicals found in permanent dyes you are trying to avoid, such as p-phenylenediamine, dihydroxybenzene, and aminophenol.

The only exception is pure henna, a vegetable dye that, in its natural state, imparts a reddish color to your hair.

To make your own ultra-safe, all-natural hair tints, try these suggestions from the laboratories at Purdue University:

- *For red highlights or to enhance red hair:* Mix ½ cup of beet juice with ½ cup of carrot juice. Pour on damp hair, and let sit for 1 hour before washing out. If you spend that hour sitting in direct sunlight (or use the heat of a blow dryer), the effects will be even more dramatic.

- *For blonde highlights:* Mix 1 cup lemon juice with 3 cups of chamomile tea that has been brewed, cooled, and strained. Pour over damp hair and let sit for 1 hour. Again, sunlight or a blow dryer will enhance the properties of the color. Wash out and follow with a conditioner. For significant blonde color, use daily for up to three weeks.

- *For brunette hair:* Prepare strong black coffee or tea. Shampoo normally, then pour the mixture through hair fifteen times, using the same liquid to rinse each time. (Do this by placing a large pasta or soup pot in the sink to catch the rinse, then pour into a large jar for the next rinse.) On the final rinse-through, leave on hair for fifteen minutes. Finish with a final rinse of clear water.

You also might want to consider that most permanent wave or straightening products have a strong odor. Since pregnancy increases your sense of smell and can make you ultra-sensitive to many scents (even those that never bothered you before), your salon appointment could cause you to lose your breakfast or lunch—and then some. Because some odors can linger on hair for up to several days, you might end up feeling more than a little queasy following your perm. All things considered, if you can avoid going without these chemical treatments, do so, at least until your second trimester.

Your Pregnancy Manicure

Besides some concern over the products you use on your hair, you may also have questions regarding nail care. This may be of particular concern, since at least some of the products commonly used in a manicure have, over the last several years, come under some scrutiny in regard to health and safety. At least some of the ingredients commonly found in nail polishes and removers—including methyl, methacrylate, and acetonitrile—are not recommended for use during pregnancy. What's more, according to the Food and Drug Administration, what goes on your nails can be absorbed into your body—and when it is, at least some of these questionable compounds can break down into other harmful chemicals, including cyanide, a deadly poison. Other ingredients in nail lacquers, such as formaldehyde and toluene, are also suspected of causing problems, and most experts agree they should be avoided during pregnancy.

The good news is there are a variety of "safe" nail products that can deliver color and shine without compromising your baby's health. Most are biodegradable, and many replace harmful chemicals with natural essential oils and herbs. Some are so safe, they're even edible. Among the most often recommended products are Almost Natural Nail Polish Remover, Sante Nail Polish, Go Natural Nontoxic Nail Polish, and Peel Off Polish. Many salons stock these products for use on their pregnant patients. Others will use whatever polish you bring, but do check with your manicurist before scheduling an appointment.

In addition, don't overlook the power of totally natural vegetable stains to add color to your fingers and toes. Boiled and concentrated beet

juice can give nails a luscious berry-color stain, as can strawberry or rasp-
berry juice. Just dip a small, clean eyeliner or eye shadow brush into the
juice and paint away, topping with a nontoxic clear coat for shine. You
can also use an all-mineral makeup product, such as Michael Maron's
Everything Powder. Buffing the colored minerals into your nails with a
cotton swab can impart a healthy pink glow. A quick zip under your nail
tips with a whitener pencil and a coat of clear, nontoxic gloss, and you
have an instant French manicure.

When it comes to acrylic nails or nail tips, surprisingly, doctors seem
less concerned. Clearly, the safety profile of any product depends a great
deal on its individual ingredients. And since there are so many types of
acrylic nail solutions on the market, it's difficult to make any general suggestions. That said, at least some medical experts contend that because so
little of this product is actually placed on your nail, you are not likely to
absorb enough to do your baby any real harm. The bottom line: There are
virtually no medical studies on artificial nails and pregnancy, so check with
your doctor and abide by what his or her experience shows to be true.

Foot Fetish:
Taking Care of Your Pregnant Tootsies

As you may have already begun to notice, the natural weight gain you experience during pregnancy alters your center of gravity—and that, in
turn, changes the way your feet bear the weight of your body. What's
more, because pregnancy can hamper circulation to your lower half, often
your feet can swell, particularly at the end of the day. All this will become
more apparent as your pregnancy progresses and your baby grows. However, that doesn't mean you won't have at least some achy foot problems
right from the start of your pregnancy—particularly if you have a job that
requires you to spend a lot of time on your feet.

Among the best ways to counter these problems is with a lavender
foot bath, which medical studies have shown can not only ease aching
tootsies, but do wonders for overall levels of stress. In research conducted
at the Nagano College of Nursing in Japan, doctors found that soaking
feet in a hot bath infused with lavender oil for just ten minutes not only
increased circulation to the feet and legs, it brought about measurable

changes in the autonomic nervous system—the area of the brain that controls stress and anxiety. The changes, say the study doctors, reflected an increased sense of relaxation. While both unscented foot baths and those infused with lavender helped increase circulation in the feet and legs, only the lavender foot baths were able to induce the state of relaxation.

TO MAKE YOUR OWN RELAXING LAVENDER FOOT BATH

Fill a foot basin or small plastic trash can with water that is warm to the touch (about 100 degrees or less). To the water add up to 5 drops of essential oil of lavender. Blend with your hand until oil diffuses through the water. Immerse both feet, and soak for ten minutes. **Important:** Remember to **never** put any essential oils directly on your skin.

For extra lavender comfort, rub feet with lavender-scented cream, such as Elaria's Extra Rich Lavender Body Cream or Johnsons' Bedtime Lotion with lavender.

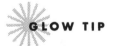 **GLOW TIP**

Cool It!

To soothe sore, swollen tootsies, fill a 16-ounce plastic soda bottle with water, and put it in the freezer. After it's frozen, roll your foot back and forth over it until the pain subsides.

Roy Corbin, D.P.M.

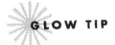

GLOW TIP

Tea Totaling Tootsies

To reduce swollen, aching pregnant feet, boil a pot of black tea, pour into a bowl, and let sit overnight. The next morning soak your feet in the cool tea for fifteen minutes. Feet will look and feel refreshed and beautiful.

Ling Chan, Ling Skin Care, New York

The Quick-Lift Peppermint Foot Massage

If time is of the essence and you're a pregnant woman on the go, go, go, then this ten-minute do-it-yourself peppermint foot rejuvenation treat is for you. While the use of peppermint is slightly controversial during *early* pregnancy, most experts agree it is safe and very effective anytime after the sixteenth week of gestation.

To begin, place 8 ounces of any nut- or fruit-based food oil (almond, olive, or sesame seed) into a clean jar. Add 3 to 5 drops of essential oil of peppermint. If your skin is very dry, you can also include a few teaspoons of wheat germ oil. Cover and shake well. Place a few drops of the oil directly on your feet. Concentrating on the soles of the feet first, use your thumbs to make small circular movements on the entire foot pad. Stroke and rotate each toe, pulling slightly, but **making certain to steer clear of the webbing between your toes.** If you have a few spare minutes, continue your massage up your leg, to your knees, always moving upward, toward the direction of your heart.

When your massage is completed, rub your feet vigorously all over with a terry-cloth towel and, if possible, elevate your legs for five minutes. You should feel an immediate increase in your circulation, a decrease in foot and leg swelling, and more energy in your step!

If you don't want to make your own peppermint foot oil, try Orjene's Peppermint Foot Cream, Belli Cosmetics Foot Relief Cream, or Magia Bella's Instant Leg Energizer.

Important Warnings About Foot Massages: Never massage directly over a varicose vein. In addition, always steer clear of the webbing between toes, and do not put pressure on the indentation between the ankle bone and the heel. Experts say pressure in these areas could encourage contractions.

Your Pregnancy Style: Some Final Words

Whether you choose to spend a great deal on your new pregnancy image or are forced to make do with only minimal purchases, it's important to remember to always allow who you are to shine through. While you may look like someone else entirely and even feel as if that little life inside you is taking over the girl you used to be, remember that what you see in the mirror is only temporary. Try to look past the image to see the you who remains inside. While how you look is an important part of your image, it's not everything. Remember, too, that in fashion, as in life, you can embrace change without losing touch with who you are.

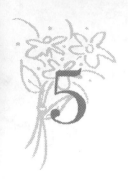

Exercising for Two

Workouts for a Healthy Pregnancy

In the not-so-distant past, the sight of a pregnant woman on a basketball or tennis court would cause quite a stir. While doctors and exercise professionals alike agreed on the benefits of exercise during pregnancy, most had a rather narrow definition of what activities that could encompass.

Not so today. Now more than ever, women are being encouraged to not only participate in pregnancy-related workouts, but also continue enjoying a wide variety of sports and other physical activities. In 2002 the American College of Obstetricians and Gynecologists embraced an updated set of guidelines that expanded the view of acceptable activities during pregnancy. In fact, most obstetricians now believe that as long as exercise is not done with an eye toward weight loss, *and* your diet can compensate for the caloric losses of working out, even strenuous activities are considered okay for some women during pregnancy. In fact, even women who never exercised before getting pregnant are now being urged to incorporate at least some form of activity in their prenatal care.

While this change in attitude was a long time in coming, the wait was not without merit. In the past decade, and particularly in the last five years, we have learned much about a woman's body and particularly the benefits of remaining active during pregnancy. Research has shown that pregnant women who *do* participate in some form of exercise generally have fewer aches and pains, better control of blood pressure and blood sugar, increased energy and less fatigue, better self-esteem, good weight control, and easier weight loss after birth. Many also experience increased stamina during labor and delivery. Some physicians, including Dr. James Clapp III, professor of reproductive biology and obstetrics and gynecology at Cleveland's Case Western Reserve University, claim that women who exercise during pregnancy also experience fewer cesarean sections and less need for forceps deliveries, episiotomies, and epidurals.

And in case you are wondering whether exercise might affect your risk of miscarriage, research shows that it won't. In another study conducted by Dr. Clapp, the rate of miscarriage was actually lower in runners and aerobic dancers than in women who stopped working out during pregnancy.

During an annual meeting of the Society for Maternal and Fetal Medicine, doctors from the Swedish Medical Center in Seattle revealed that women who are physically active in their first and second trimesters are 34 percent less likely to develop preeclampsia, a dangerous form of pregnancy-related high blood pressure. The study reported that even routine activities performed during pregnancy, such as taking the stairs instead of an elevator, can substantially reduce risks.

As good as physical activity can make *you* feel, it can also help your baby—reducing birth complications and even some birth defects. At least one study showed that babies born to active mothers had decreased levels of fetal distress both before and during labor. Even more astounding: These babies also experienced improved neurodevelopment right from birth. At least one study with a five-year follow-up found that babies born to mothers who were physically active during pregnancy had advanced neurodevelopment clear through the age of five. These babies were smarter and more advanced than those born to sedentary moms.

Staying in Shape: What to Expect from Your Pregnant Body

As important as it is to remain active and fit, doing so is not without some concerns. "If you continue to train while pregnant without understanding the contraindications for exercise, you can seriously jeopardize your own health as well as that of your [baby]," says fitness expert and certified trainer Brad Schoenfield, CSCS, CPT.

The fact is, from almost the moment you conceive, your body begins changing—and those changes can figure heavily into what activities you will be able to perform comfortably *and safely.* Among the most important of those changes is a difference in the way your cardiovascular system responds to physical exertion, beginning right at the start of your pregnancy.

Those changes begin with a temporary shortage in the amount of oxygen-carrying red blood cells, which occurs in the first trimester. This can leave you with less energy and working a little harder to meet the same exercise goals as you did before pregnancy. As your uterus begins to grow, it pushes against your diaphragm—the large muscle that lies just between your chest and abdomen. As a result, your breathing becomes more rapid *and* more shallow, which can also cause you to feel more out of breath than ever before. And it may take you longer to catch your breath after working out.

These are all changes you need to expect and acknowledge, along with the realization that you should not be seeking to break any exercise records during pregnancy—especially your own. Although part of you may be psychologically fighting the change in how your body looks and feels, resist the temptation to compare yourself to how fit you were before pregnancy. Instead, set new standards of achievement and new goals to reach while baby is in tow. Your goal should be to maintain a fitness level you feel good about so you can withstand labor and recover from childbirth as quickly as possible.

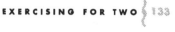

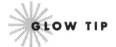 **GLOW TIP**

Get Motivated

Before you start exercising, always wash your face and rinse with cool water. Doing so will energize you and create a fresh state of mind. Even if you don't feel like exercising, convince yourself to do just five minutes; after that, if you don't want to continue, then you can stop.

Karen Voight, fitness expert and celebrity coach

The Heart of Your Workout Routines: Cardiovascular Changes

In addition to changes in breathing, during pregnancy your cardiovascular system itself is undergoing adjustments that can affect your activity level. First, your heart rate will be naturally faster during pregnancy, even when you are relaxing. And it won't return to the resting rate as quickly after exercise. Depending on how fit you were prior to conception, during pregnancy it could take fifteen minutes or more for your heart rate to return to its resting level after working out. Keeping these facts in mind can help you to plan your fitness activities and know what to expect from your body.

One of the most significant cardiovascular-related changes of pregnancy occurs sometime around your fourth month. At this point your uterus will have expanded so much that lying flat on your back for any significant length of time could result in a compression of the vena cava, a major vein that carries blood back to your heart. When compressed, this low-lying vein will cause your heart to beat more slowly, which in turn can result in dizziness. It can also interfere with blood flow to your uterus, which in turn can make it difficult for your baby to receive important nutrients, including oxygen. The American College of Obstetricians and Gynecologists cautions that, beginning in the twentieth week of pregnancy, you should refrain from participating in *any* fitness activity that causes you to lie flat on your back.

In addition, your heart rate and blood flow to your baby can both be affected if you stand motionless in one position for any extended period of time—something that is sometimes required in certain yoga postures or when doing certain isometric exercises. Thus, you may need to adjust some workout routines to accommodate these changes as well.

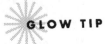

GLOW TIP

Perfect Posture

Pregnancy puts pressure on your back, so protect yourself from the extra weight by always thinking "perfect posture!"

- Balance your weight around the center of gravity in your lower spine and pelvis.

- Remember to hold your head erect, without pushing the chin forward.

- Always keep your shoulders back and down.

- Maintain the normal curves of your back. Stretching exercises will help.

- Change your position often. Don't wait until your back is aching.

- Relax. Take deep breaths. This will force your chest upward.

- Don't ever stand with your knees locked. Keep your joints loose.

Denise Austin, fitness expert and author

The Beach Ball Effect: How Your Size
Affects Your Fitness Activities

Depending on what trimester you are in right now, you may have already noticed some pretty significant changes in the shape of your body—not only in the size of your growing tummy, but also your breasts. What many women don't realize is that the larger their breasts get during pregnancy, the greater their risk of injury to ligaments, particularly if they are doing any impact exercises, such as aerobics or running.

One solution is to make certain to wear a sports bra during exercise and, as your belly grows, to consider a pregnancy girdle or "tummy sling" when working out. This can help you avoid both pulled muscles and ligaments and a hernia. In fact, the more support you can give your body while working out, the lower your risk of injury, particularly to your breasts and stomach, where you are likely to experience the most profound changes.

For many women, however, the most disconcerting thing about the change in size is the accompanying change in the center of gravity, a problem that affects your sense of balance. Since balance is key to preventing sports injuries, it's something you clearly can't ignore. This is particularly true if you plan to participate in any activity that relies heavily on balance to avoid injury, such as downhill skiing or horseback riding. You should also note that even a slight decrease in your sense of balance can increase your risk of sprains and strains during any activity that involves quick movements, such as tennis or racquetball, for example. You must always consider whether or not your center of gravity is affected, and if so, how much, before deciding which activity is right for you at any given time during your pregnancy.

Along with your increasing size comes an increase in the production of a hormone known as relaxin. As its name implies, its purpose is to relax cartilage, which is extremely helpful during labor and delivery. For many years, nearly all doctors believed the increase in relaxin levels during pregnancy increased the risk of sports injuries, mostly by relaxing the supporting joints and muscles so much that turning an ankle or twisting a knee out of joint was more likely. More recently, however, some researchers have begun to question this logic. Among the newest thoughts is that relaxin's only effect may be on the cartilage surrounding the *pelvis* and lower back, where it works to help the passage of baby's head through the birth canal. Joints and ligaments in other parts of the body may not be affected.

What nearly all experts do agree on, however, is that the excess weight of pregnancy increases pressure on your joints—and that, combined with a decreased sense of balance can increase your risk of joint, muscle, and even bone injury during exercise. That's something you're going to have to keep in mind as you plan your fitness activities.

The Heat Is On:
Pregnancy and Your Body Temperature

Among the physiological changes of most concern during pregnancy are those involving body temperature. Sobering statistics reveal that excessive body heat, particularly during the first trimester, can dramatically increase your baby's risk of birth defects, particularly those affecting the brain and spine. In at least one study published as early as 1992, researchers from the University of North Carolina at Greensboro found that when a woman's body temperature rises above 102.5 degrees during the first twelve weeks of pregnancy, her baby's risk of spina bifida—a life-threatening defect involving spine formation—increases significantly.

Likewise, in animal studies conducted by the U.S. Environmental Protection Agency, it was learned that when body core temperature increases by as little as a few degrees above normal, offspring can suffer skeletal malformations, particularly rib and vertebra defects. The animals subjected to increased body temperature also gave birth to fewer live offspring. Since exercise normally raises body temperature, this information is of major concern for any woman who remains physically active during pregnancy.

That said, other, more recent research has suggested that pregnant women may have a built-in temperature resistance mechanism that protects their bodies from dramatic increases during physical activity. And, studies have also revealed that pregnant women who exercise regularly may simply be more efficient at dissipating body heat during exercise, because they begin sweating at a much lower body temperature.

Until additional research resolves the debate, most experts suggest

Real Life

WATER AND PREGNANCY FITNESS

Q: I've heard that if you drink enough water just prior to exercise, you can keep your body from overheating. Is this true? And if so, how much water should a pregnant woman drink and when: before, during, or after exercise?

A: One of the key dangers in overheating is dehydration—a problem that can have dramatic effects on your pregnancy. One way to prevent dehydration is to ensure adequate fluid intake, particularly water, before, during, and after exercise. But how much fluid do you need? Generally, two 8-ounce glasses of water for every sixty minutes of exercise, or 8 ounces for every thirty minutes of working out is recommended.

However, experts from the American College of Sports Medicine believe that pregnant women must make a bit more effort. They recommend drinking two glasses of water about two hours before beginning a workout and then consuming between 5 and 12 ounces more every fifteen to twenty minutes during physical activity.

One easy way to see how much water you need to consume *after* working out is to use your scale as a guide. Because most immediate weight changes following exercise are due to water loss, the American College of Sports Medicine experts say to weigh yourself before and after each workout session, then drink two glasses of water for every pound you've lost. That should help ensure proper hydration.

One more clue: Use the color of your urine as a guide. When you are properly hydrated, your urine should be almost colorless or very pale yellow. The darker it turns—from a deep yellow to a "beer" gold—the greater your risk of dehydration and your need for more water.

you play it safe and monitor your body temperature during heavy physical activity, particularly when you begin to feel overheated. If your temperature is starting to climb—the danger point is about 101 degrees—slow down and cool down. Then make whatever changes in your fitness activities are necessary to prevent overheating in the future.

Your Active Pregnancy:
What's Safe, What's Not

Because every pregnancy is different, and every woman's personal health profile is strictly her own, what's right for one pregnant woman may spell disaster for another. That's why only your personal obstetrician is qualified to advise you on the best and safest physical activities for you.

That said, there are a number of activities that doctors universally agree on as being generally safe and recommended during pregnancy. These include:

Swimming (no diving)

Riding a stationary bicycle

Walking

Kegel exercises

Low-impact aerobics

Water aerobics

Stretching and toning

Tai chi

Participation should last around thirty minutes and take place up to five days a week. If you want to exercise longer—up to sixty minutes a day— make sure to discuss it with your doctor.

There are also some activities that doctors generally believe are *unsafe* to do during pregnancy or that should be done using extreme caution. The sports to avoid: any involving a high risk of falling or abdominal trauma, including:

⊘ Downhill skiing

⊘ Gymnastics

⊘ Horseback riding

⊘ Water skiing

⊘ High-impact aerobics

⊘ Bicycling on uneven terrain or wet pavement

⊘ Jogging on uneven surfaces or wet surfaces

⊘ Scuba diving

⊘ Inline skating

⊘ Ice skating

According to BabyCenter.com fitness expert Jill Stovsky, during pregnancy you should also avoid deep-knee bends, full sit-ups, and lunges, since all three can strain ligaments and lead to an increased risk of tears in the pelvic region.

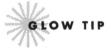

GLOW TIP

Talk It Out!

The best way to ensure that you are not overdoing a pregnancy workout is to do a "talk test." If you can talk comfortably while you are doing your workout, you are exercising at a reasonable level.

Denise Austin, fitness expert and author

Getting Physical:
Making Workouts Safer for You and Baby

As long as you have your doctor's approval, you may be able to continue at least some, if not all, of the fitness activities you participated in before pregnancy. Oftentimes, however, there will be a few changes you'll have to make in your routines, particularly to help guard against injuries. To this end, here is a list of good-sense modifications. These are changes you should consider making to your workout routines during pregnancy. However, do keep in mind that these modifications are for women who were already actively involved in these sports *before* getting pregnant. If you have never participated in these activities, experts say it's probably not a good idea to start during pregnancy.

- *Ballet:* Because joints and ligaments may be looser, avoid overly strenuous moves, such as kicks, splits, leaps. Use the barre if balance becomes an issue.

- *Boxing classes:* Don't box with another person, use punching bag training only; drink lots of extra water during circuit-training classes; watch balance.

- *Cross-country skiing:* Avoid hills; don't ski at elevations over 10,000 feet.

- *Dance aerobics:* Switch from high- to low-impact moves.

- *Golf:* Don't carry your own golf bags; alter your swing when necessary to accommodate belly and breasts.

- *Hip-hop dance classes:* Reduce the intensity of your workout and get your doctor's okay on a new target heart rate; perform low-impact moves only, keeping one foot on the floor at all times; avoid jumping, stepping side to side, and quick turns.

- *Karate classes:* Don't work with a partner; practice moves solo; avoid hyperextension of knees, hips, elbows, and shoulders; don't do any moves that feel uncomfortable or cause pain.

- *Softball:* Avoid positions that involve body contact or squatting for long periods (catcher); no sliding into bases.

- *Step aerobics:* Lower step by up to six inches and avoid jumps.

- *Tennis:* Play singles with a partner who is less skilled than you are; play doubles with a partner who is more skilled than you are.

- *Treadmill:* Lower speed if you find you can't talk normally or are out of breath while walking.

- *Volleyball:* Avoid continuous jumping; don't take dives for low balls.

- *Weight training:* Avoid the Valsalva maneuver (forcefully exhaling without releasing air) and walking lunges; use lighter weights and do more repetitions; don't use weights lying flat on your back.

- *Yoga:* Avoid extreme positions, holding one position for extended period of time, back bends, belly poses; perform standing poses using a chair, or stand next to a wall for extra balance; avoid any poses that place stress or strain on your abdomen.

Running and Pregnancy: Some Special Advice

In the past, there was so little information on the effects of running during pregnancy that most doctors simply advised their patients to avoid it. Not so anymore. In fact, a study conducted by a fitness and health research organization, the Melpomene Institute, showed that pregnant runners averaging 24.8 miles per week, three months prior to conception, were able to give birth to healthy, full-term babies. Some 80 percent of the women had vaginal births, and their babies each weighed an average of seven pounds, six ounces.

As a result of this and similar studies, doctors have opened their minds to the idea that, for many women, running is a viable exercise during pregnancy. You may even be able to run until well into your third trimester—as long as you have your doctor's okay. Do, however, make doubly certain not to skip on warm-ups, particularly stretching. Because joints and ligaments may be less predictable during pregnancy, you need to take extra steps against injury in large muscles like hamstrings and quadriceps, as well as your Achilles' heel and your lower back. Stretching can offer you that protection, as can making certain that you run only on smooth, flat pavement.

In addition, make certain you listen to your body and modify the intensity, speed, and frequency of your runs depending on how you feel.

Real Life

PILATES AND PREGNANCY

Q: I love to do Pilates. It seems like a gentle exercise to me, but a friend says it may not be safe to do during pregnancy. Is there any information on this—and if it is safe, are there are any precautions I should take?

A: Pilates is a form of exercise that concentrates on strengthening the abdominal muscles and increasing circulation—both of which can be a real bonus during pregnancy to you and your baby. The key, however, is to know which Pilates moves are safest and best and which ones need to be modified or even avoided during pregnancy. Certainly an exercise that causes you to lie on your back—as many Pilates routines do—should be avoided beginning in the twentieth week of pregnancy. You should also avoid extreme rotational movements of the spine (there is a small chance they could disrupt the placenta) and positions and movements that challenge your balance and increase the risk of falling.

According to Mari Winsor, a world-recognized Pilates trainer and authority, you should always check any exercise routine with your doctor first. Once he or she gives you the okay, then, says Mari, follow a video, find a pregnancy-specific book, or get some instruction on the best Pilates moves for pregnancy. If you've never done Pilates before, it's important that you get some kind of hands-on training if you are going to begin this form of workout during pregnancy.

Stop the minute you feel any contractions, even harmless Braxton-Hicks contractions, which are a normal part of pregnancy. Likewise, stop if you feel any ligament pain, and, of course, when you are tired or if you experience any cramps or bleeding.

Experts say that later in pregnancy, you should cut your workout regimen, reducing the amount of time you run, the distance, and the speed. Many women report cutting back mileage by 40 percent in the second trimester and up to 70 percent in the third trimester. As your pregnancy progresses, think about doing less running and adding more cross training

An Expert's Opinion on

SPINNING IN CYCLES

One of the more popular ways to work out on an exercise cycle is spinning—riding your bike with the same kind of intensity used while racing. While you might not be going anywhere in terms of distance, spinning definitely sets your metabolism flying. Although there is little evidence either for or against spinning during pregnancy, one small study had encouraging results. Fifty women who participated in spinning three to five times a week during pregnancy, with a target heart rate of 150 to 160 during exercise, fared well, with no complications. However, unless you have been an avid bike rider and racer, pregnancy is probably not the best time to try spinning. If you have been spinning prior to getting pregnant, it's probably okay to continue—as long as your doctor says it's fine.

to your regimen. In fact, most experts agree that the closer you get to your delivery day, the fewer impact activities you should do—switching instead to things like riding a stationary bike or swimming. If your doctor approves, you may be able to do these activities right up until your water breaks.

Health Clubs, Personal Trainers, and Pregnancy

If you are like many women, you may already be a member of a health club or even working under the guidance of a personal trainer. In many instances, both scenarios can be beneficial in helping ensure you remain active during pregnancy.

There are, however, a few precautions you need to take and a few things to remember. First, regardless of how skilled, athletic, or charming your personal trainer may be, if he or she is not trained in pregnancy workouts, you may not receive the best advice. While many personal trainers have degrees in physiology *and* knowledge about exercise and pregnancy, some have little more than their own experience upon which to draw. So, as soon as you know you are pregnant, check to see if your trainer is qualified to instruct you at this time—and be sure to ask for specific credentials. You might also want to inquire about any other pregnant clients the trainer has worked with, and ask if you can speak to one or two. Don't be afraid of insulting your trainer—most will welcome your inquiries.

This same advice is doubly important if you are working out in a health club and utilizing on-site personnel for advice and help. Also, check with health club management about any regulations regarding pregnant women using the facilities. Some may require a doctor's note saying it's okay that you exercise.

Also ask if they have any programs or instructors who are specifically trained to work with women during pregnancy. Even if you consider yourself a workout expert, you'll gain many benefits from a class that focuses not only on the kinds of exercises you need during pregnancy, but also on the safety boundaries to keep your body healthy and strong with a minimal risk of injury. In many instances, fitness programs are offered at the hospital where you deliver, so check with your doctor at the start of your pregnancy.

Regardless of where you work out, or who is advising you on what to do and how to do it, always apply an extra dose of common sense, and don't participate in any activity unless your doctor says it's okay. In addition, if you feel you are being worked too hard, tell your trainer or class leader—and make certain she or he is aware of the safety guidelines featured later in this chapter.

In addition, if you are working out at a health club during your pregnancy, forgo some of the perks membership may offer, such as saunas, hot tubs, and Jacuzzi or whirlpool baths. Besides safety issues involving heat, hygiene can also be a concern at some fitness centers, where it can be easy to pick up a dangerous intimate infection even while sitting around a hot tub or sauna. The same may be true of showers and dressing rooms. So, if you aren't overly impressed by a health club's cleanliness, limit your activities there to working out, and leave bathing for when you get home.

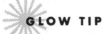

"I remained active throughout my pregnancy, but I was careful—just walking and prenatal yoga," says supermodel **Cindy Crawford**.

For actress **Catherine Zeta-Jones**, playing lots of golf was her primary exercise. She says she stepped up the heat after baby Dylan was born with "cardio workouts and toning sessions with a fitness guru."

Superstar **Madonna** reports she kept in great shape during her second pregnancy with baby Rocco by practicing "power yoga and Pilates"—also the choice of actress **Liz Hurley**. Madonna reports she also did lots of walking and cycling through pregnancy and postpartum recovery—and got her buffed and toned body back rehearsing for a new world tour.

MTV's **Jenny McCarthy** kept in shape by spending four days a week on a treadmill or power walking, and two days doing free weights.

Working Out for Pregnancy Health: What to Do

In addition to helping you enjoy a more comfortable pregnancy, prenatal exercise can also pay off when it's time to deliver your baby. According to experts from the University of Michigan (UM) Health System, stretching and toning specific muscles in your abdomen, pelvis, and back while you are pregnant can help you get through labor and delivery more easily and possibly with less pain. There is even some evidence to show that exercises you do *while* pregnant can make it easier to get your body back in shape after your baby is born.

To help you accomplish all this, what follows is a special Pregnancy Exercise Guide. Based on the newest fitness guidelines from the American College of Obstetricians and Gynecologists, and featuring advice from experts at the University of Michigan, it can help you to personalize a pregnancy workout program that is right for you. If you've done little or no exercise prior to conceiving, these guidelines can serve as a great starting point. If you're already a fitness buff, they can help spotlight the new moves you need to add to your regular workouts to help ensure you achieve flexibility in the muscles specific to pregnancy and delivery.

Of course, regardless of your fitness level, always check with your doctor before starting this or any exercise program. Be certain to let your physician know both the type of workout you plan to do, how long each session will last, and how many times a week you plan to exercise.

Your Pregnancy Exercise Guide: Workouts That Work!

WORKOUT #1: THE KEGEL

What It Does: Stretches and conditions muscles supporting pelvic organs, including your bladder and uterus. During and after pregnancy, Kegel exercises can help prevent incontinence; during delivery strong pelvic muscles can help reduce the risk of tearing the perineum (the area between the vagina and the anus) and help facilitate an easier birth.

Before You Start: It's important to isolate the muscles that are involved in this exercise. To do this, try stopping and starting urine flow while going to the bathroom. The muscles you use to stop urine flow are the muscles that are involved in the Kegel exercise.

An alternate approach: While sitting or lying down, insert a finger in your vagina and squeeze your vaginal muscles until your finger feels the pressure.

How to Do It: Once you have isolated the muscle group, the exercise itself consists of tightening, holding, then releasing these muscles in cycles of five to ten seconds as many times a day as possible. To help remember to do them, pick an activity that you do several times a day—such as an-

An Expert's Opinion on

GOING BEYOND THE KEGEL

For registered nurse Bonnie Rote, mastering the Kegel exercise is important. But Rote takes the Kegel concept one step further with something called neuromuscular disassociation. As director of the Women's Exercise Programs at Pasack Valley Hospital in Westwood, New Jersey, Rote teaches women to contract and tighten a *single* group of muscles while relaxing all others. How can this help? During delivery, she says, you will have to "work" your uterus, while the rest of your body relaxes. So, knowing what it feels like to contract one muscle group while relaxing all others can help prepare you for delivery. To learn the skill, Rote says try clenching your fist while relaxing all the other muscles in your body. While it's going to take a bit of concentration, once mastered, you should be able to transfer to your uterus the feeling of tightening just one muscle group and relaxing the rest.

swering the phone or sitting at a traffic light—and always do your Kegels at the same time.

The Kegel Plus: Sit on the floor cross-legged; pull up your vaginal muscles (as if you are stopping the flow of urine); release the muscles *slowly,* pushing until you feel a slight bulge in the area between your vagina and anus. Relax to the count of five and repeat. Five to eight repetitions a day can go a long way in helping to condition these muscles.

Workout Hints: Don't bear down or squeeze your thighs, back, or abdominal muscles. Breathe slowly and deeply. Squeeze to the count of four and relax to a count of five. Try to do this for five minutes at least once a day.

WORKOUT #2: THE TAILOR SITTING AND TAILOR PRESS EXERCISES

What It Does: Conditions the muscles of the inner thighs and the pelvic floor muscles, plus helps to release tension in the thoracic spine.

How to Do It: For the Tailor Sitting: Sit on the floor, bring your feet close to your body, and cross your ankles (a cross-legged position). Feel the muscle pull as you try bringing your legs as close to your trunk as possible. Hold this position as long as you can, then relax.

For the Tailor Press: Sit on the floor, bring the bottoms of your feet together so that the soles are touching, and pull your legs as close to your body as possible. Place your hands under your knees and use the muscles in your legs to push down, using your hands to resist the pressure. Count to three slowly, and release. Gradually increase your number of knee-hand presses until you can do ten twice a day.

WORKOUT #3: THE TAILOR STRETCH

What It Does: Strengthens the lower back and increases flexibility.

How to Do It: Sit on the floor with your back straight and legs out-stretched in front of you, about a foot apart, with ankles turned outward. Begin by stretching your arms toward your left foot, then back; reach to the center, then back; reach to the right, then back. Move slowly and don't bounce, holding each stretch for several seconds. Gradually increase your stretches until you can do ten rounds twice a day.

WORKOUT #4: THE PELVIC TILT

What It Does: Strengthens pelvic muscles and eases back pain.

How to Do It: While standing, tighten your abdominal muscles and hold; while holding, tighten your buttocks by squeezing and pulling under. Hold for a few seconds, keeping knees relaxed. Release and start again. Work up to ten tilts twice a day.

Real Life

EXERCISE AND BELLY SPLITS

Q: I recently read that the muscles of your belly can actually split apart during pregnancy, particularly if you exercise your stomach too hard. Is this true? If so, what are the signs and is it dangerous?

A: The problem you are referring to is called diastasis—a slight separation of the two halves of a muscle known as the *rectus abdominis*, which runs down the center of your belly. The problem primarily occurs in the process of making room for your growing uterus. And while it is not an unusual occurrence, it's not extremely common either—and exercise generally does not play a role in whether or not it occurs.

If diastasis does develop, it may not be as easy to spot as you might think. While in some women it can be obvious—they can touch the muscles on top of the abdomen and actually feel the separation—in others it's hardly visible at all. But whether or not you feel it or see it, doctors say it's not something you need to be worried or concerned about. Shortly after giving birth, the two halves of this muscle come together without consequence. (See Chapter 12 for information on how diastasis can play a role in exercising after delivery.)

WORKOUT #5: THE PELVIC ROCK

What It Does: Strengthens pelvic muscles and increases flexibility; provides abdominal support, relieves low-back pain; helps baby move through the birth canal.

How to Do It: Get down on hands and knees, positioning your hands directly under your shoulders and your knees directly under your hips. Inhale deeply. While exhaling slowly, pull your abdominal muscles inward and tighten your buttocks, arching your back into a C shape. As you hold this position, perform a Kegel, tightening pelvic muscles; hold for several seconds and relax, allowing back to go straight. Repeat eight times.

Exercise Safety: What You Need to Know

Whether you are participating in an organized sport or simply performing pregnancy-specific exercises, there are some safety concerns you need to keep foremost in your mind. Indeed, in January 2002 the American College of Obstetricians and Gynecologists convened a special committee to help establish pregnancy-specific safety guidelines that would ensure the health of both active mothers and their babies.

Among the most important suggestions was to ensure that calorie intake remains high during pregnancy. Their specific recommendation: that you consume at least 300 calories a day over and above your normal dietary intake, and that you eat more if heavy physical activity is burning up what you do eat. They also caution against any physical activity performed for the purpose of weight loss or weight control during pregnancy.

In addition, you should not participate in heavy physical activity during pregnancy if you suffer from heart and lung disease, or if you have been diagnosed with any of the following pregnancy-related problems:

Incompetent cervix / cerclage

Multiple pregnancy

Persistent second- or third-trimester bleeding

Placenta previa (after twenty-six weeks)

Preeclampsia

Premature labor

Ruptured membranes

You should also talk to your doctor about modifying your workouts if you suffer with severe anemia, chronic bronchitis, or poorly controlled high blood pressure or high blood sugar; if you are either extremely underweight or overweight; or if you led an extremely sedentary lifestyle before getting pregnant.

Finally, terminate activity immediately and call your doctor if any of these problems occur anytime during exercise:

Vaginal bleeding

Dyspepsia (heartburn) prior to exertion

Dizziness or faintness

Headache

Chest pain

Muscle weakness

Calf pain or swelling (until blood clots can be ruled out)

Preterm labor

Decreased fetal movement

Amniotic fluid leakage

Blurred vision (can be a sign of dehydration)

Irregular heartbeat (skipped beats or very rapid beating)

Pelvic pain or significant pain of any kind

Strong uterine contractions

Any vaginal fluid leaks

Most often problems will be temporary, and you will be able to resume your workout at a slightly slower pace. However, only your doctor can tell you that for sure, so don't make the decision on your own!

GLOW TIP

Get Ready for Exercise

Decide ahead of time what workout tape you want to use, place it in the VCR, and set it to the beginning of the warm-up. When it's time for your scheduled workout, you'll be glad that you need only push a button to begin. Remember that a balanced fitness program includes upper and lower body conditioning, aerobic activity, and flexibility training.

Karen Voight, fitness expert and celebrity trainer

A Final Word: It's Never Too Late to Start

For those of you who participated in fitness activities prior to conception, exercising throughout pregnancy is not likely to present many challenges. Although you may have to make some adjustments in your workout regimes and maybe add a few pregnancy-related moves to your fitness program, as long as you are healthy, it's likely your doctor will give the okay to continue doing most if not all of your previous activities.

Many of you reading this book, however, may not have much of an aerobic background. Maybe you never exercised at all prior to conception—or your activities were minimal or sporadic. If power-shopping through the grocery store twice a week pretty much sums up your total fitness regime, then you know what I'm talking about.

If you didn't participate in many fitness activities prior to conception—and especially if you didn't exercise at all—remember that it's never too late to start. A 1990s study conducted by the University of Miami found that women who didn't start exercising until they were well into their second trimester *still* improved their fitness levels dramatically. When they began the program, they could last only five minutes on a treadmill before their heart rate kicked into overdrive. But by the fifteenth week of participating in a simple walking program, they could stay on the treadmill more than twelve minutes before their heart rate peaked. Even with the extra weight of pregnancy, they were able to accomplish some significant fitness goals. By comparison, the control group—who didn't do any exercise during the fifteen weeks—actually lost strength and stamina, experiencing a decrease in cardiovascular endurance.

Which brings me to a final point: If you haven't exercised much before conception, and particularly if your workouts were sporadic, it's important that you take it slow and that you get some guidance in starting your pregnancy fitness program. Besides taking your doctor's advice, it's important to get some input from the fitness world. For many of you, the ultimate smartest move you will make is to enroll in a prenatal fitness class. With instructors who are specially trained in the fitness needs of pregnant women as well as the limitations of the pregnant body, you can be assured that you are not only working out safely, but also working out correctly.

Chances are your obstetrician probably knows of a few local instructors and classes, and often community centers or libraries have information as well. You might also want to check with the hospital where you plan to deliver your baby—many have on-site prenatal workout programs that can help get you started.

Finally, don't overlook the Internet as a great source of pregnancy fitness advice and information. Websites such as www.Fitfor2.com, www.FitPregnancy.com, and www.BabyCenter.com are teeming with expert advice on how to develop a pregnancy fitness program that's right for you.

The point is, don't be ashamed to ask for help or to admit that you haven't been exercising in the past. Everyone will admire your decision to do so now—and you're likely to find plenty of support.

6

Pickles, Candy Bars, and Pizza for Breakfast

Nutrition and Your Pregnancy

From virtually the moment you conceive, your baby depends on you for everything—every building block of *his or her* life begins with *your* life. Thus, the foods you eat become your baby's sole supply of energy, protein, vitamins, minerals, and all nutrients necessary not only to sustain life, but to grow and develop. As *your* blood volume expands to accommodate your pregnancy, and your body prepares to store protein and other types of calories in anticipation of nursing, your own nutritional needs increase as well.

So it's safe to assume that regardless of what your nutritional requirements were before pregnancy, they are somewhat higher now—and they may continue to increase until your baby is born. That's just one of the many reasons why a prenatal diet plays such a critical role not only in the growth and development of your baby, but in how you feel throughout your pregnancy.

Because each of us has an individual appetite as well as individual preferences for the foods we like to eat, no one prenatal diet is right for every pregnant woman. However, there are *some* important nutrients that experts say *must* be included in your daily diet—factors that will not only help your baby grow, but can help keep *you* healthy and strong as well.

To this end, what follows is a guide to the ten most important nutrients you will need throughout your pregnancy. Based on recommendations from the American College of Obstetricians and Gynecologists, as well as the advice of New York University Medical Center's senior clinical nutritionist Samantha Heller, MS, RD, it can help you intelligently plan meals that will not only suit your palate, but increase your strength and help your baby grow.

Top Ten Pregnancy Nutrients: What You Really Need

1. *Protein.* As the main building block for your baby's growth and development, protein helps in the manufacture of new cells and produces the extra blood you need, as well as extra energy stores, for labor and delivery. Protein is also essential for the production of hormones and enzymes and for regulating fluid balance.

   Amount You Need: At least 60 grams per day: at least three meals daily consisting of 2 to 3 ounces of a protein source at each meal.

   Best Sources: Lean red meat, poultry, seafood, eggs and beans, soybeans, tofu.

2. *Carbohydrates.* An immediate source of energy on which you can draw for the tasks at hand, carbohydrates also supply the energy necessary for your baby to develop and grow.

   Amount You Need: About 9 servings daily from the high-fiber group and 3 to 4 from fruits and vegetables—equaling approximately 60 percent of your daily calorie intake.

   Best Sources: High-fiber carbohydrates such as whole-grain breads and fortified whole-grain cereals, brown and wild rices, potatoes and pasta, as well as fruits and vegetables.

3. *Calcium.* Providing the mineral content for your baby's teeth and bones, calcium also keeps your muscles strong and healthy during pregnancy. When your intake is low, your baby pulls calcium from your body stores and eventually from your bones. Keeping your intake high ensures baby's needs are met without tapping into your reserves. Medical literature suggests adequate calcium intake during pregnancy may also minimize muscle spasms and leg cramps as well as help retain proper fluid balance in your body.

Amount You Need: 1,200 milligrams daily.

Best Sources: Low-fat dairy products, including milk, cheese, yogurt, and ice cream; soy milk; calcium- and vitamin D–fortified orange juice; as well as spinach, sardines (with bones), and salmon.

4. *Iron.* This nutrient is needed to ensure a good supply of red blood cells, which transport oxygen to your baby. Iron also helps bring oxygen to your own muscles and organs, thus minimizing pregnancy fatigue.

Amount You Need: 30 milligrams daily.

Best Sources: Lean red meat, spinach, whole-grain breads and cereals, kidney beans and other legumes, and fortified cereals.

5. *Vitamin A.* A nutrient necessary to form your baby's tooth enamel and hair, vitamin A also aids in the growth of the thyroid gland, and is important for good eyesight.

Amount You Need: Up to 100 micrograms daily retinol equivalent or 5,000 international units (IUs). **Note:** Vitamin A can reach toxic levels via supplements, but rarely from food sources.

Best Sources: Carrots, dairy, leafy greens, sweet potatoes.

6. *Vitamin C.* This contributes to the development of your baby's skin, tendons, and bones through the formation of collagen. Since collagen breaks down when your skin is stretched during pregnancy, keeping vitamin C levels high may also help guard against the formation of stretch marks as your belly grows.

Amount You Need: 70 to 80 milligrams daily.

Best Sources: Citrus fruits, broccoli, tomatoes.

7. *Vitamin B6.* This vitamin aids baby's overall development and may help reduce your risk of morning sickness in the first trimester. A deficiency during pregnancy may increase your risk of edema (swelling) and high blood pressure and increase your baby's risk of cleft palate. This nutrient will also help your body to utilize protein, carbohydrate, and fat more efficiently. It also plays a role in protein and fatty acid metabolism, as well as helping to produce red blood cells.

Amount You Need: 2.2 milligrams daily.

Best Sources: Green leafy vegetables, navy beans, baked potatoes, watermelon, soybeans, salmon, beef, liver, pork, ham, whole-grain cereals, bananas.

8. *Vitamin B12.* Necessary for the development of your baby's red blood cells, vitamin B_{12} also reduces the risk of oxygen deprivation, which in turn can reduce the risk of some birth defects. For you, B_{12} protects the nervous system and increases your ability to produce red blood cells.

Amount You Need: 3 to 4 milligrams daily.

Best Sources: Liver, meat, fish, poultry, milk. Since this nutrient is found only in animal foods, vegetarians need to get their supply via supplements.

9. *Fat.* Necessary as a source of long-term energy for you, your baby also needs some fat to grow.

Amount You Need: Fats should make up about 30 percent of your daily caloric intake, with a low intake of saturated fat and cholesterol, and eliminating as much trans fat (hydrogenated) as possible.

Best Sources: Plant oils such as canola, safflower, peanut, and olive. Remember to also count fats you get from meat, dairy, nuts, peanut butter, margarine, and salad dressings.

10. *Folic Acid.* One of the most important nutrients for pregnancy, folic acid not only helps make the extra blood cells needed to sustain your pregnancy, it can dramatically reduce your baby's risk of serious birth defects of the skull and spine—and could save his or her life. A study published in March 2002 in the journal *Lancet* found that mothers who took both folic acid and iron supplements during pregnancy also reduced their baby's risk of developing childhood leukemia. A study published in the *Journal of the American Medical Association* in October 2002 found that folic acid deficiency was linked to increased risk of miscarriage, but that taking supplements could help women avoid that risk. (See "An Expert Opinion on Folic Acid and Pregnancy Loss.")

Amount You Need: 400 micrograms daily. If you have had a previous child with a spine or skull defect, you may need up to 4 milligrams daily during the first three months of your current pregnancy.

Best Sources: Spinach, collard greens, turnip greens, romaine lettuce, broccoli, asparagus, whole-grain bread and cereal, strawberries, oranges, pinto beans, black beans, lima beans, chickpeas.

Your Pregnancy Appetite: What to Expect

Knowing what foods you should be eating during pregnancy is one thing; including them in your diet may be another matter entirely. The reason is your pregnancy appetite, which, from almost the moment you conceive, can undergo some dramatic and even confusing changes. While at certain times you may feel ravenously hungry, other times you may have almost no appetite at all.

This situation may be particularly true at the start of your pregnancy, a time when many women first develop food aversions—a sudden, often mystifying intolerance of certain tastes and smells, sometimes even of meals they just couldn't live without before. For some women, the first undeniable sign of pregnancy is an extreme intolerance of the smell or taste of foods they used to adore. While your particular food aversion could include almost any dish, among the most common are the taste or

An Expert Opinion on

FOLIC ACID AND PREGNANCY LOSS

As important a nutrient as folic acid is, particularly in decreasing the risk of neural tube defects, earlier research suggested that this important gain might be offset by an increased risk of miscarriage in the first trimester— an increase that, at the time, researchers believed was caused by folic acid supplementation. However, in October 2002, a study published in the *Journal of the American Medical Association* laid these fears to rest. The report, a major collaborative research effort between doctors from the National Institute of Child Health and Development (NICHD) in the United States and those from the Karolinska Institute in Sweden, revealed that not only was folic acid supplementation safe to use during pregnancy, it actually *prevented* miscarriage. The study also showed that folic acid did not increase the risks of miscarriage, as previously thought, but that women who miscarried were not taking enough of it to reap the protective effects.

"Our findings suggest that there is now a true potential for reducing the risk of miscarriage . . . and that there are other benefits to taking folic acid, other than reducing the risk of neural tube defects," says Dr. James L. Mills, chief of the NICHD pediatric endocrinology branch.

smell of coffee, particularly fresh perked, as well as fried foods, alcohol, and creamy or rich sauces or desserts.

For the most part, doctors believe that hormones are behind pregnancy-related appetite changes. More specifically, because both estrogen and progesterone can heighten your sense of smell and taste, as their levels climb they can cause a kind of sensory overload. In essence, some smells and tastes can seem so powerful, they become intolerable, sometimes even triggering the nausea and vomiting of morning sickness (see Chapter 1).

And while neither food aversions nor morning sickness are considered harmful in early pregnancy, they can begin to cause problems if they interfere with your ability to eat nutritiously, or even eat at all. A National Institutes of Health study published in the *American Journal of Obstetrics and Gynecology* in August 2001 found that going thirteen or more hours without food during pregnancy caused elevations in corticotropin-releasing hormone (CRH), a biochemical that has been linked to preterm labor. The women who experienced prolonged periods with no food during pregnancy were the most likely to deliver premature babies.

If nausea or food aversions keep you from eating during early pregnancy, do talk to your doctor. You may also want to try some of the remedies for morning sickness featured in Chapter 1, which can help control nausea. Remember, even small amounts of food are better than no food in early pregnancy.

UNDERSTANDING YOUR FOOD CRAVINGS

As you head toward your second trimester, you might notice that food aversions are suddenly taking a backseat to food cravings—strong, even overwhelming desires to gulp down any number of different foods, sometimes in what can seem like rather bizarre combinations. For some women, these desires can become so strong, they can't get to sleep or even relax until they have the food they crave. Some of the more offbeat foods pregnant women have reported craving include pickles wrapped in cheese, salsa right out of the jar, steak fat, black olives on Sara Lee Cheesecake, Cheez Whiz sandwiches, eggplant pizza, and root beer candies.

In a survey of some 20,000 women conducted by BabyCenter.com, it was noted that 40 percent of pregnant women craved sweets, particularly ice cream, while 33 percent craved salty, greasy treats like potato chips. Just 17 percent couldn't get enough spicy Mexican food, and a mere 10 percent wanted health foods like citrus fruits or green apples.

While no one really knows what's behind food cravings, many believe that a deficiency of nutrients may drive us to eat what our body lacks. According to San Diego midwife and herbalist Cindy Bilew, a craving for red meat may be our body's cry for more protein, while urges to eat bushels of peaches, for example, may signal a need for more beta carotene, which is found in high amounts in this fruit.

Real Life

CHOCOLATE BARS AND PREGNANCY RISKS

Q: I'm an absolute candy-holic—I love candy bars and always ate them before pregnancy. Now that I'm pregnant, my habit has grown worse— I can't stop eating them. My doctor said they are dangerous for me and my baby and told me I have to stop. Is this true: Can a chocolate bar really harm my pregnancy?

A: An occasional chocolate bar, or even several a week, is not going to do you any harm, particularly if you are eating an otherwise healthy diet. Your doctor's concerns, however, are on target. First, your sugar cravings could mean you are at increased risk for insulin resistance and possibly gestational diabetes—problems that can affect your baby's health and endanger your life as well. (See Chapter 1.) Additionally, studies published in August 2001 in the *American Journal of Obstetrics and Gynecology* found that when a lot of your daily caloric intake is made up of foods high in sugar (like most chocolate bars) and polyunsaturated fats (also found in some candy bars), you increase your risk of the dangerous, pregnancy-related blood pressure problem known as preeclampsia. (See Chapter 1.) So, you probably should think about at least reducing the number of candy bars you eat, seeking satisfaction in a few bites rather than a whole bar.

Because, however, it can be hard to believe we lack the nutrients found in supermarket cheese spread or a bag of fried corn doodles, other research shows that our nutrient deficiencies may simply be influencing our taste buds. This, in turn, may be what is driving us to certain foods— even though these foods may not be linked to the nutrient we are missing. Many alternative-medicine doctors, for example, believe that a craving for chocolate is triggered by a lack of B vitamins, despite the fact that chocolate itself is not a strong source of this nutrient.

A similar idea is behind the theory about why certain pregnant women develop a condition known as pica—bizarre cravings for nonfood items, such as clay, ice, starch, and cigarette butts. In many instances, these cravings occur in women who have iron deficiencies, even though there is no iron in any of these substances.

Most experts believe the reason behind food cravings is the same as the one behind food aversions: in a word, hormones. According to nutritionist Elizabeth Somer, the extreme hormonal changes that occur during pregnancy are likely to play the biggest role in determining what we want to eat. Because our sense of taste and smell can become so exaggerated during pregnancy, Somer says that certain foods simply taste better, so we want more of them.

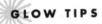

GLOW TIPS

Celebrity Moms on Food Cravings

Rock-and-roll diva **Toni Braxton** coproduced and recorded a record album while pregnant with her first child, who was born on Christmas Day. Her pregnancy cravings: "First it was Doritos and applesauce; then cheese pizza, but I had to dip the pizza in French dressing; now I'm into Kellogg's Frosted Mini-Wheats," said Toni in an interview during the second trimester of her second pregnancy.

During her second pregnancy, rock idol **Madonna** reportedly whiled away the hours munching on olives and eggs. And for supermodel **Cindy Crawford**, it was "bean burritos from Taco Bell on a daily basis," which she says fulfilled her pregnancy cravings.

For MTV's **Jenny McCarthy**, French fries and chocolate made her pregnancy heart sing! "A batch of Duncan Hines brownies every night!" says McCarthy.

TO INDULGE OR NOT TO INDULGE:
HOW TO HANDLE FOOD CRAVINGS

Depending on what foods you crave during your pregnancy, experts say you can indulge a little—or a lot. Certainly if you're craving yogurt and fruit shakes, or bowls of oatmeal, you probably can eat to your heart's content without any problems. If, however, your cravings are more apt to lead you to the bakery and not the health food store, you must exercise some moderation, particularly if you are concerned about losing those extra pregnancy pounds after giving birth. While it's okay to eat the foods you crave *once in a while*, give in only when the craving hits hard and nothing else seems to satisfy you. Also try not to eat what you're craving on an empty stomach. If you do, you're likely to eat a lot more of it. You should also never allow yourself to feel hungry—one reason to keep a lot of healthy snacks on hand. In addition, never skip breakfast. Studies show that food cravings can be much more intense if you skip your first meal of the day.

You can also try eating a small portion of the food you crave and waiting twenty minutes. You may be surprised to discover that the craving goes away with little more than a taste. If, after twenty minutes, you want more, allow yourself another small portion, and wait twenty more minutes. For most women, doing this can cut the amount of the craved food by about half—saving half the calories.

Finally, if you exercise a little culinary creativity, you can satisfy your craving with more healthy fare, such as fruit instead of ice cream, or a whole-wheat bagel instead of a doughnut. (See "Healthy Food Fixes.")

But what if all you can think of is that premium high-fat strawberry ice cream? Experts say concentrate on what it is about this snack that's making you feel satisfied. Is it the sweet taste, the creamy consistency, the strawberry flavor? Or maybe it's just the idea of eating something cold that satisfies those cravings. Once you lock in on the nature of what you crave, substituting a low-calorie, somewhat healthier food may be easy: perhaps eating strawberry sorbet, low-fat strawberry yogurt, or fresh strawberries with a low-fat dessert topping instead of ice cream.

HEALTHY FOOD FIXES FOR
YOUR PREGNANCY CRAVINGS

If You Crave	Try Eating
Ice cream	Nonfat frozen yogurt, sorbet, or sherbet
Cola	Mineral water with fruit juice or a slice of lemon or lime
Doughnuts/pastry	Whole-grain bagel with fruit jam
Cake	Low-fat banana or zucchini bread
Sugar-coated cereal	Whole-grain cereal or oatmeal with brown sugar
Potato chips	Baked, low-sodium, low-fat chips, popcorn, or pretzels
Sour cream	No-fat sour cream or nonfat plain yogurt flavored with herbs
Sundae toppings	Fresh berries or bananas
Canned fruits in heavy syrup	Fresh fruit, frozen unsweetened fruit, fruit packed in water or juice
Lunch meats	Low-fat or fat-free versions; substitute turkey or soy bologna or hot dogs for the beef variety
Whipped cream	Ice-cold no-fat milk whipped with a handheld immersion blender

Important Note: If you are one of a small number of women craving nonfood items during your pregnancy, including clay, starch,

Real Life

PASTA, PREGNANCY, AND
LOW-BIRTHWEIGHT BABIES

Q: I read somewhere that eating a lot of pasta during pregnancy can be harmful to your baby. I'm very concerned about this because I'm six weeks' pregnant and find that pasta is the only food I can tolerate—which works out pretty well, because I love it! But now I'm worried that I might be harming my baby. Is pasta bad for pregnancy?

A: In itself, pasta is not harmful to you or your baby. In fact, if you eat a whole-wheat variety, it can add important fiber and other nutrients to your diet. That said, studies published in the *British Medical Journal* as early as 1996 found that a diet high in carbohydrates and low in protein in early pregnancy appeared to suppress the growth of the placenta, thereby reducing the level of nutrients your baby receives. Moreover, when combined with a reduced intake of dairy and meat proteins later in pregnancy, a high-carbohydrate diet further stunted the growth of the placenta, and low-birthweight babies resulted. Conversely, another study published in the same journal said the high-carbohydrate theory applies only to women who are malnourished to begin with—those who are extremely thin prior to getting pregnant.

As far as *your* pasta-eating habits are concerned, if possible, switch to a high-protein variety and incorporate some dairy or meat into each dish you make. For example, top pasta with mounds of grated cheese, or try an Alfredo sauce using fresh cream to combine dairy and protein. Tossing a meatball or two onto the plate can help—or if that doesn't seem appetizing, serve your pasta with meat sauce. As long as your carbohydrate intake does not exceed the recommended 60 percent of your daily caloric intake, indulging your pasta fantasies should be fine.

wood, or anything not considered a food, do not give in to your craving and see your doctor immediately.

Putting on the Pregnancy Pounds:
What You Need to Know

Once upon a time, doctors believed that the more weight a woman gained during her pregnancy the healthier her baby would be. Not so anymore. Today doctors know that excessive weight gain will increase your risk of gestational diabetes as well as high blood pressure, endangering both your life and that of your baby.

A Scandinavian study of more than 600 women published in the journal *Obstetrics and Gynecology* in 2002 found that excessive weight gain increased the risk of preeclampsia as well as a series of labor and delivery problems. The study also found that problems increase in direct proportion to how much extra weight you gain. For example, research shows that women who gain up to forty-five pounds during pregnancy have triple the rate of health problems of those who gain just thirty-four pounds.

TOO SKINNY FOR A HEALTHY PREGNANCY?

As dangerous as gaining too much weight can be, doctors also recognize that not gaining enough weight, particularly early in pregnancy, can also increase certain risks for you and your baby. In research conducted in 2002 at the Baylor College of Medicine in Houston, Texas, Dr. Laura Goetzel and colleagues studied over 900 pregnant women, only to find that those who gained the least amount of weight during pregnancy had the most birthing complications—even more than those who overate and gained too much. The undereaters also had nearly three times the rate of premature birth when compared to women who overate, and slightly more than two-thirds the rate of normal eaters. Ultimately, the underweight women gave birth to babies weighing nearly 400 grams (14 ounces) less than women who gained excess weight or those who gained the correct amount.

A second study conducted at St. Mary's Hospital in London and published in June 2001 found that women with the lowest body mass index (BMI) during pregnancy delivered nearly twice as many low-birthweight babies as women who were of normal weight. Even the Scandinavian study mentioned earlier found that women who gained too little weight during their pregnancy had almost as many complications as those who gained too much.

PERSONALIZING YOUR PREGNANCY WEIGHT GAIN

In the past, doctors routinely suggested that all women gain about twenty-four pounds during their pregnancy. That figure, the result of a report released in 1970 by the U.S. National Research Council, was considered the norm for more than twenty years.

But by 1990, however, thinking began to change. The National Academy of Sciences Institute of Medicine began revising the guidelines, suggesting instead that pregnancy weight gain be determined by a woman's prepregnancy body mass index—her measurement of body fat prior to conceiving. Today most doctors suggest that women with a high BMI, who carry extra fat stores before pregnancy, gain less weight than those who have a normal or a low BMI prior to conception.

Recently, researchers have also begun to consider the importance of a woman's ethnic background when charting a pregnancy weight profile. A study published in a recent issue of the *Journal of the American Dietetic Association* called attention to the fact that a woman's body shape and composition of body fat can vary greatly among different ethnic groups— so much so that recommendations for one group may not apply to another.

And with the popularity of fertility treatments and the boom of multiple births, some researchers believe that even more "wiggle room" is needed when determining proper weight gain for women carrying twins or triplets. The latest studies suggest that the more babies you are carrying, the more you need to eat, and the higher your pregnancy weight should be.

But it's not only the amount of weight you gain that's important; *when* in your pregnancy you gain that weight matters as well. While in the past doctors believed that you could easily get through your whole first trimester without adding an extra pound—and that it was even okay if you lost weight—now that philosophy has also begun to change.

In studies published in July 2002 in the *American Journal of Clinical Nutrition,* Professor Judith E. Brown of the University of Minnesota showed how weight gained during the first trimester was directly linked to a baby's birthweight, even more so than pounds gained later in pregnancy. Her research showed that every kilogram (2.2 pounds) a woman gained during her first trimester translated into a 31 gram boost in baby's birthweight. What's more, gains seen in the third trimester had virtually no influence on baby's size at birth. Therefore, Brown believes that there is a distinct "window of opportunity" to maximize your baby's growth with your own weight gain, and that window is clearly in the first trimester. Babies who don't gain enough weight during gestation have an increased risk of a variety of health problems, including learning disabilities that may follow them clear into adulthood. Today even the American College of Obstetricians and Gynecologists recommends that you gain between three and five pounds during your first trimester.

But how much weight should you expect to add during your *entire* pregnancy? According to the American College of Obstetricians and Gynecologists, make note of your prepregnancy weight, then use this chart to determine how much to gain.

Prior to Pregnancy	What to Gain During Pregnancy
Underweight (BMI less than 20)	28 to 40 pounds
Normal weight (BMI 20 to 25)	25 to 35 pounds
Overweight (BMI 26 or more)	15 to 25 pounds

In addition, guidelines published in 2000 by the American Dietetic Association suggest that mothers carrying two or more babies can gain up to 50 pounds during their pregnancy.

Real Life

WHERE DOES THE WEIGHT GO?

Here's where your average pregnancy weight gain goes:

Baby: 7.5 pounds

Reserved energy stores: 7 pounds

Extra blood volume: 4 pounds

Total body fluids: 4 pounds

Amniotic fluid: 2 pounds

Breasts: 2 pounds

Uterus: 2 pounds

Placenta: 1.5 pounds

If you gain a healthy amount of weight during pregnancy, giving birth should automatically cause you to lose up to twenty pounds.

Five Pregnancy Super Foods— and Why You Need Them

Besides eating the proper amount of calories every day, what you eat matters too. A number of new studies have shown there are important benefits to be gained from including certain pregnancy "super foods" in your diet. From protecting against high blood pressure and preeclampsia, to reducing your baby's risk of birth defects and early delivery, including just a few key items in your weekly diet can help round out your nutrition requirements while supplying some of the nutrients necessary for a healthy pregnancy. Here are the foods the experts say you should consider.

SUPER FOOD #1: ALL-BRAN CEREAL
WITH EXTRA FIBER

Because it's packed with dietary fiber, which studies show may reduce your risk of preeclampsia, this cereal tops the list of pregnancy must-haves. In research conducted by Dr. Ihunnaya O. Frederick of the Swedish Medical Center in Seattle, Washington, women who ate some 24 grams of fiber a day saw a 51 percent reduction in preeclampsia compared to women who ate just 13 grams of fiber a day. Plus the extra fiber you get from this cereal can reduce constipation, which in turn may help you avoid another pregnancy complication—hemorrhoids.

A serving of Kellogg's All Bran with extra fiber contains a whopping 13 grams—plus a full 400 micrograms of folic acid. Along with fruits and grains like apples and brown rice, you can easily reach your fiber quota without a calorie overload. Other good-for-you, high-fiber cereals include Quaker Oatmeal, Kashi Good Friends, General Mills Rice Chex, and Kellogg's Raisin Bran. One caveat: If you don't regularly eat a lot of fiber, take it slow. Start with a third of a cup of cereal and slowly work your way up to a full serving over several weeks.

SUPER FOOD #2: ORANGE JUICE

Drink just two cups of orange juice a day and you could reduce your blood pressure by up to 10 points, say doctors from the Cleveland Clinic Foundation—a critical drop if your pressure is high during pregnancy. The high C content may also reduce your risk of preeclampsia (see below). In addition, if you take your prenatal vitamin with orange juice or any other vitamin C–rich food, it will aid in iron absorption and may reduce constipation problems associated with iron supplements. If you choose an orange juice fortified with calcium, available from Minute Maid and Tropicana brands, you'll be giving yourself an additional nutritional boost that's good for you and your baby.

SUPER FOOD #3: BANANA STRAWBERRY SMOOTHIE

Packed with key vitamins and nutrients, this drink (made by combining strawberries, bananas, and low-fat milk, soy milk, or yogurt in a high-speed blender) could help you avoid premature labor. Studies conducted by Dr. James Woods Jr. at the University of Rochester School of Medicine and Dentistry showed that high levels of vitamin C and E—higher than what is found in prenatal vitamins—could prevent the premature rupture of membranes during pregnancy, which reduces the risk of premature labor. A second study published in the July 2002 issue of the journal *Epidemiology* found that women who consumed higher amounts of vitamin C during pregnancy cut their risk of preeclampsia nearly in half. Keeping calcium levels high may also help control fluid retention, which in turn can decrease your risk of high blood pressure.

SUPER FOOD #4: SALMON

Studies conducted by renowned Danish professor of obstetrics Dr. Niels J. Secher showed that the long chain N-3 fatty acids found in salmon and other oily fish can reduce the risk of premature birth. In studies published in the *British Medical Journal* in 2002, Secher and his colleagues showed that women who ate less than 15 grams of fish daily (equal to 0.15 grams of fatty acid) had the greatest risk of premature delivery. But you don't have to eat a lot of fish to get the important protection. The study also found the risk of premature birth fell from 7.1 percent in women who ate no fish during pregnancy to just 1.9 percent in those who ate just one fish meal a week.

And if you want your newborn baby to sleep like . . . a baby, eating fish while you are pregnant may help. A study published in the *American Journal of Clinical Nutrition* in 2002 found that babies of mothers who ate fish-based fatty acids during their last trimester had healthier sleep patterns in the first few months after birth. The key, say experts, is a fatty acid known as DHA (docosahexaenoic acid). Abundant in cold water fish, such as trout or salmon, it is essential to the development of a baby's brain and central nervous system. When levels of DHA are inadequate, your baby's nervous system may not fully develop, which in turn can disrupt sleep patterns. But be careful not to overdo fish consumption, as mercury levels in some varieties can be high. Six to twelve ounces each week is considered safe. (See "Pregnancy and Food Safety" later in this chapter.)

SUPER FOOD #5: LOW-FAT YOGURT

Among the more obvious pregnancy benefits of low-fat yogurt is its high calcium and protein content, with little or no fat. High calcium not only helps your baby grow a strong skeleton, it also helps reduce muscle cramping in you—and when levels are adequate, it may even help you control bloating and water retention. But apart from its calcium value, medical literature also suggests that eating up to 8 ounces of yogurt daily may help reduce your risk of yeast infection—a common pregnancy problem. While there is no absolute proof that eating yogurt will help, a number of anecdotal reports suggest that it can offer some protection.

Prenatal Vitamins:
Are You Taking the Right One?

Although your diet should supply many of the nutrients both you and your baby need, there is no question that prenatal vitamins also have a place in your pregnancy. Whether you choose to take a prescription vitamin or purchase one over-the-counter, the high levels of nutrients and the formulations in most of these products can prove extremely beneficial to both you and your baby. Although some women have problems taking prenatal vitamins (they can cause stomach upset, heartburn, indigestion, and nausea), oftentimes switching brands, changing the time of the day you take your vitamins, and watching what you eat right before or right after can help.

Unfortunately, however, not all prenatal vitamins are created equal— and even though you take them religiously, you could end up with substantially fewer nutrients than what is printed on the label. The reason has to do with what chemists call the "dissolution factor." This is the rate at which a vitamin pill must break down in your stomach in order to be properly absorbed and utilized by your body. While the dissolution factor affects all nutrients, at greatest risk is one of the key vitamins essential for the health of your pregnancy: folic acid.

The reason is that folic acid is absorbed in your upper intestines just after it passes from your stomach. If dissolution of your vitamin tablet is too slow—taking an hour or more to dissolve—your body misses the window of opportunity to absorb this nutrient. Instead, it passes from your upper to lower intestines, where it is passed from your body without ever being fully absorbed. Going down the drain as well is the protection you thought you were gaining from your vitamin. This is precisely what researchers from the University of Maryland proved was happening with nine popular prenatal vitamin products. In studies published in 1997, Stephen Hoag, Ph.D., and colleagues revealed that only three out of nine over-the-counter prenatal formulations they tested had dissolved soon enough for adequate absorption. Two of the nine products tested released less than 25 percent of their folic acid content in that first hour.

Because vitamin formulations often change, the researchers declined to mention the names of the vitamins tested, and have kept their specific results secret. However, if you're thinking of moving over to a prescription formula—just to play it safe—think again. In research published in *Advances in Therapy* in July 2002, another group of researchers compared seven popular prescription prenatal vitamins and found only three met the standards for folic acid dissolution. Only one vitamin—Prenate Advanced—had what was considered a high level of folic acid dissolution. On average, the researchers found that the first-hour dissolution rate for four of the prescription products tested ranged from 38 percent all the way down to 0 percent. And the study authors claim their results corroborate other research showing a vast difference in the dissolution rate of prescription prenatal vitamins.

IS YOUR VITAMIN UP TO SNUFF? HOW TO TELL

According to the U.S. Pharmacopeia (an agency that tests and then sets voluntary dissolution standards on vitamins), to be effective, a vitamin tablet must release 75 percent of folic acid content within one hour of hitting your stomach. And you can put your own vitamin to the test, right in your own kitchen.

To Do the Test: Drop your vitamin tablet into ½ cup of vinegar and stir gently. Every five minutes or so, give it another stir. Within twenty minutes, your vitamin should be completely broken down—if not dissolved, at least separated into tiny particles. If it is not, says Hoag, the dissolution rate should be questioned, and he advises that you choose another brand, repeating the test until you do get the proper dissolution rate. This same test should be done both on vitamin pills you swallow whole and on chewable vitamins, which also must undergo some dissolution once they hit your stomach. If you *are* testing a chewable vitamin, you might want to try crushing it into pieces similar to what would happen if you chewed it before putting it in the vinegar solution.

While some doctors are keenly aware of a vitamin's dissolution rate and are able to suggest those that are up to snuff, don't be surprised if your obstetrician is less familiar with this than you expect. Many doctors are not as aware of nutritional updates as they could be, so on this issue, you may be on your own.

Pregnancy and Food Safety: What You Must Know

Over the last several years, a number of significant food dangers have come to light—some of which have presented serious, even life-threatening problems for pregnant women and their babies. While some of these problems have come from the foods themselves, at other times food preparation practices have caused the difficulties.

Because of the tremendous publicity many of these events received, pregnant women were often left feeling as if the neighborhood grocery store or even the local deli was a glaring den of danger. In reality, however, there is really only a short list of food safety concerns you need to observe during your pregnancy.

For most experts, fish tops the list, including both saltwater and freshwater varieties. According to the Environmental Protection Agency

(EPA), mercury levels in many types of fish can damage a baby's brain and central nervous system, particularly when that fish is consumed in large quantities.

In 2002 the National Academy of Sciences issued a stern report stating that levels of mercury contamination allowed by the Food and Drug Administration (FDA) were still too high for pregnant women. Perhaps not coincidentally, in July 2002 an advisory panel to the FDA recommended that pregnant women and women of childbearing age also limit consumption of tuna, at least until more in-depth mercury studies are completed.

What to eat right now: Experts say limit freshwater fish to no more than 6 ounces weekly; total fish consumption should be limited to 12 ounces per week. Meals to avoid completely include tile fish, swordfish, king mackerel, and shark.

One more caveat: Many obstetricians also suggest that patients avoid eating sushi (raw fish) during pregnancy. While the fish itself is not necessarily a problem, sushi does carry a higher than normal risk of a bacteria that causes an infection known as listeria—which, as you will read in just a few minutes, can be very dangerous for you and baby.

The Caffeine Controversy: What You Should Know

First they said it was okay; then no amount was safe; now moderation seems to be the key. The controversy is over the use of caffeinated products in pregnancy, including not only coffee, but also colas, chocolate, and, to some extent, even tea. While some studies clearly showed links between caffeine and miscarriage, particularly early in pregnancy, others found the opposite, and cited caffeine-laden beverages as safe.

What doctors do agree on, however, is that caffeine intake does affect your baby. The reason, say experts from the March of Dimes, is that caffeine crosses the placenta—meaning it gets into your baby's body. Because your baby's system is not yet mature enough to break down and eliminate chemicals the same way your body can, blood levels of caffeine may remain higher longer. Some studies have shown that excessive caffeine intake during pregnancy can increase baby's heart rate and respiration considerably, and may cause him or her to spend more time awake in the days and nights directly following birth.

The bottom line: *Moderate* caffeine consumption is okay during pregnancy, with most doctors agreeing that 150 milligrams daily—or about one and a half cups of coffee—is not likely to increase your risk of miscarriage or cause your baby problems. The Organization of Teratology Information Service is slightly more liberal, suggesting that three cups of coffee, or a total of 300 milligrams of caffeine daily, is fine.

More recently, studies published in the *American Journal of Epidemiology* in April 2002 pushed the caffeine envelope even further. Here very precise studies on nearly 900 pregnant women revealed that consuming up to 500 milligrams of caffeine daily (about 22 ounces of brewed coffee) is not likely to cause any problems.

So, how much caffeine is okay for *you* to consume? The best advice is talk to your doctor. Discuss the latest research and be sure to get your obstetrician's opinion on what's considered safe during *your* pregnancy. In the meantime, however, if you are consuming a lot of caffeine-rich products, it makes good sense to cut back as much as you can, beginning as early in your pregnancy as possible.

When deciding what foods to limit, researchers from McGill University in Canada warn not to forget about the "hidden" caffeine in many foods—items you might not necessarily think of as being caffeine-rich. To help you stock a healthier "pregnancy pantry," here are a few foods with some eye-opening and surprising caffeine levels. You can see how they stack up against more common caffeine-rich foods such as tea, coffee, and chocolate, which are included at the end of the list.

Food	Caffeine Content
Celestial Seasonings Iced Lemon Ginseng Tea (16 oz)	100 mg
Bigelow Raspberry Royale Tea (8 oz)	83 mg
Snapple Ice Tea—all flavors (16 oz)	42 mg
Coca-Cola Classic (12 oz)	34.5 mg

Dr. Pepper (12 oz)	42 mg
Mountain Dew Soda (12 oz)	55.5 mg
Ben & Jerry's No-Fat Coffee Fudge Frozen Yogurt (1 cup)	85 mg
Starbucks Coffee Ice Cream (1 cup)	40–60 mg
Häagen-Dazs Coffee Ice Cream (1 cup)	58 mg
Dannon Coffee Yogurt (8 oz)	45 mg

Common Caffeine-Rich Foods and Beverages

Hershey's Special Dark Chocolate Bar (1.5 oz)	31 mg
Cocoa/hot chocolate (8 oz)	5 mg
Brewed coffee (8 oz)	135 mg
Instant coffee (8 oz)	95 mg
Designer coffees (8 oz)	
Orange Cappuccino	95 mg
Café Vienna	90 mg
Cappuccino Mocha	60–65 mg
Swiss Mocha	55 mg
French Vanilla/Irish Creme	50 mg
Viennese Chocolate Café	25 mg
Decaffeinated Coffee— all flavors and regular (8 oz)	3–6 mg
Black tea—leaf or bag (8 oz)	50 mg
Green tea—leaf or bag (8 oz)	30 mg

Real Life

ARTIFICIAL SWEETENERS AND BIRTH DEFECTS

Q: Is it safe to use products containing aspartame (Equal, Nutrasweet) during pregnancy? I had heard they can cause birth defects. If they are not safe, are any other sweeteners okay to use?

A: The two main artificial sweeteners—aspartame and saccharin—have been studied extensively and, despite repeated rumors of problems, have never been positively linked to any adverse pregnancy outcomes. According to research published in the journal *Seminars in Reproductive Health*, there has been "no significant relationship between the consumption of the chemical sweetener aspartame and fetal malformations or spontaneous abortions." Although only animal studies have been done, even when pregnant rats were fed huge amounts, no adverse effects were seen. Animal studies on saccharin also proved it was safe to use during pregnancy. However, don't be surprised if your doctor continues to caution against the use of these artificial sweeteners, as well as newer ones like acesulfame-K. Most medical experts concur that the fewer chemically altered substances you put in your body during pregnancy, the better off you will be.

A Final Thought:
A Little Food Safety Goes a Long Way

As important as it is to eat a healthy diet during pregnancy, it's also important to remember that even the healthiest foods can make you sick—particularly when they are not prepared or stored properly. And while a food-related illness is never a pleasant experience, it can be particularly troublesome during pregnancy, increasing health risks for both you and your baby.

Among the more devastating is toxoplasmosis—a condition that can dramatically increase your baby's risk of birth defects, particularly if you get sick during your first trimester. Caused by a parasite that lives in the intestines of cats, sheep, cattle, and pigs, it can make its way into your body when you eat raw or undercooked meat or eggs or when you come in contact with the feces of an infected animal. That's one reason doctors often advise against cleaning a cat's litter box during pregnancy, since it's easy to inhale the parasite when dust from the litter box blows into the air. According to the March of Dimes, toxoplasmosis can also end up on unwashed fresh fruits and vegetables if they are grown in a soil contaminated by an animal that carries the parasite.

A second bacteria, known as listeria monocytogenes, causes a form of food poisoning known as listeria—a disease that can dramatically increase your risk of miscarriage, stillbirth, and premature birth. You can contract listeria if you eat even small amounts of food contaminated with this bacteria, which likes to live on raw fruits and vegetables as well as processed meats, soft cheeses, and particularly unpasteurized milk products. Raw fish, in the form of sushi, can also be easily contaminated. And because listeria bacteria is a very hardy germ, contamination can be lurking on countertops or refrigerator shelves that held the tainted food.

While for many years this bacteria was seen primarily in Europe, early in 2000 it began showing up in the United States. In the fall of 2002, New York City and some other major urban areas experienced a small but significant outbreak of listeria that was traced to deli meat.

A third bacteria capable of causing food poisoning is salmonella, which can turn up in something as innocent as homemade potato salad that's been left out of the refrigerator too long. It also is readily found in raw fish used to make sushi or dishes containing undercooked eggs or poultry. When contracted during pregnancy, salmonella can be passed to your baby, sometimes with life-threatening complications.

Still another foodborne pathogen is *Escherichia coli (E. coli)*, which is common in undercooked ground beef or sausage. In large amounts, *E. coli* infection can threaten your pregnancy.

To avoid contact with foodborne pathogens and to protect yourself and your baby from harm, the National Centers for Disease Control advises pregnant women to:

- Thoroughly cook all meats and keep raw meats separate in your refrigerator.

- Wash all vegetables and fruits thoroughly before eating.

- Avoid unpasteurized dairy products.

- Avoid soft cheeses such as Camembert, brie, blue-veined cheeses, and Mexican-style cheeses.

- Avoid or reduce consumption of cold cuts, particularly deli-counter foods.

- Wash hands and utensils using hot water and soap after handling any raw food.

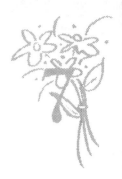

Pampering Your
Body, Mind, and Spirit

Overcoming Stress, Sleep Problems,
and Pregnancy Fears

Cell phones ringing, beepers calling, traffic, long commutes, work deadlines, and housework piled sky high. It's called stress—and it's a fact of modern living that can dramatically affect our health. Depression, anxiety, headaches, backaches, stomachaches, even colds and flu can all develop or become worse when we are under chronic stress. Add pregnancy to the mix, and experts say your health stakes can rise even higher.

The important thing to remember, however, is that even the most stressful events don't have to get your pregnancy down. While we often can't change what's going on in our world, we *can* change our reaction to it—and, in doing so, short-circuit many of its negative effects. Later in this chapter you'll learn some important new ways to turn down the volume of stress in your life and protect both your health and that of your baby. But right now it's important to learn a little bit more about how and why stress can affect your health and complicate your pregnancy.

The Stress Response:
What You Need to Know

From almost the moment you experience a stressful event, an area of your brain known as the hypothalamus kicks into high gear. It produces a chemical known as corticotropin-releasing hormone (CRH), which kicks off its own cascade of biochemical responses. The end result is a phenomenon doctors call the "stress response," which your body experiences in a number of ways. From an increase in your heart rate to a tensing of your muscles, to changes you don't even see or feel, the effects actually take place body-wide.

While short-term stress usually won't cause you any serious or long-term harm, the situation can change when even low-level tension and anxiety become chronic—particularly during pregnancy. A Finnish study published in the April 2000 issue of the journal *Obstetrics and Gynecology* reports that women under extreme stress during pregnancy are three times more likely to develop preeclampsia—the leading cause of maternal mortality.

According to Dr. Calvin Hobel, chairman of obstetrics and gynecology at Cedars-Sinai Medical Center in Los Angeles, continuously high levels of stress hormones can even affect your immune system, increasing your risk of uterine infections linked to premature labor.

How Stress Affects Your Baby

If you experience significant stress during pregnancy, it's not just your body that is affected; your baby is affected as well. High CRH levels prompt the release of yet another chemical called prostaglandin, a hormone that can trigger uterine contractions and, in the process, increase your risk of miscarriage. Moreover, the longer your stress response continues, and the more CRH your body produces, the greater that risk becomes. In studies conducted as early as 1995, researchers from the California Department of Health Services revealed that the risk of miscarriage is up to three times higher for women who experience severe stress early in their pregnancy.

And when it comes to stress, *timing is everything*: When in your pregnancy you experience anxiety makes a difference, with your first trimester the most susceptible to trouble. As your pregnancy progresses, a combination of hormones and other natural chemicals kicks in to form a kind of biological defense system that protects you and your baby, even during the most difficult and anxious moments. But during your first trimester, no such protection is in effect.

This fact was well documented in studies conducted by the University of California at Irvine following the massive 1994 northern California earthquake. In this instance, women who were in their first trimester when the quake hit were far more likely to deliver prematurely than those who were further along when the disaster occurred. Many doctors caring for pregnant women in New York City and Washington, D.C., following the events of September 11, 2001, say they saw similar reactions among their own patients. "There is a critical period during pregnancy in which the mother is most susceptible to stress," writes earthquake study researcher Dr. Laura Glynn. For many women, that is the first trimester.

But if you're thinking that it's just major events and global stresses that can affect you, think again. Studies show that the kind of stress that seems most detrimental to pregnant women and their babies involves the daily irritants that most of us face on a regular basis. Indeed, studies show that when small but chronic stresses keep CRH elevated during the first trimester, your body reprograms your labor alarm, and it rings a lot earlier than it should. You won't necessarily have a miscarriage, but you could deliver prematurely, and your baby may have a low birthweight. In a study published in the journal *Family Planning Perspective* in 2000, researchers found that women who simply admitted feeling very stressed by their lives during pregnancy were one and a half times more likely to deliver a very-low-birthweight baby—under 1,500 grams, or less than 3.5 pounds. "Stress plays a major role in early labor and in low birthweight, which are two leading causes of infant death," says Dr. Charles J. Lockwood, chairman of obstetrics and gynecology at Yale University School of Medicine.

An Expert's Opinion on

ANXIETY AND HYPERACTIVE CHILDREN

While every mother-to-be experiences some degree of pregnancy-related anxiety, those who are swept away by these emotions may, in fact, be setting the stage for their baby to be born with an anxious personality as well. In new studies conducted by Professor Vivette Glover of Imperial College in London, women who reported having extreme anxiety attacks during pregnancy and who spent much of their time panicky or scared were twice as likely to give birth to a hyperactive child. These studies were among the first to suggest that there was a chemical component to what was previously thought of as a genetic or environmental problem. "If the mother is very anxious, she changes her chemistry, [including] her hormone levels," reports Glover. At least one of those hormones—cortisol—can cross the placenta and may affect baby's developing brain. If you are feeling very anxious, Glover advises, "Take time out—talk to people, talk to a friend, talk to your [doctor]—try to do something that you feel relaxes you." Most important, she says, is to remember that even if you are extremely anxious during your pregnancy, it's not a guarantee that your baby will be affected. "Nine out of ten children of even the most anxious mothers are still perfectly okay," says Glover.

STRESS AND BIRTH DEFECTS: IMPORTANT NEWS

Among the most important new studies on stress and pregnancy are those that link high anxiety to an increased risk of birth defects. One such study of more than 3,500 women published in the journal *Lancet* in 2000 found that babies born to women who were stressed were up to 80 percent more likely to have malformations of the head, face, skull, palate, teeth, nose, eyes, ears, throat, and heart. A similar finding was documented again in a study published in the *Journal of Health and Social Behavior* in early 2002.

In addition, in 2002 researchers from Ohio State University reported that when extreme stress occurs between the twenty-fourth and the twenty-eighth week of pregnancy, your baby can experience a dramatic increase in the risk of autism—a neurological disorder that can affect the ability to learn, to talk, or even to communicate. "These are major stressors we are talking about—like the death of a loved one, the loss of a job, or something extremely traumatic that occurs specifically during these weeks of the pregnancy," says lead study author Dr. David Beversdorf, assistant professor of neurology at the Ohio State University Medical Center. And, while many factors can enter into the equation, Dr. Beversdorf is sure that when the timing of particular stressful events meshes with certain developments in your baby's brain, autism is far more likely to occur.

Overcoming the Effects of Stress: What You Can Do

While we can't always control the personal stresses in our life, we can exert power over the way in which we respond—and studies show that doing so may help you control many of the negative effects. One way to do just that is to remain as optimistic as you can during your pregnancy. How can this help?

According to the University of Pittsburgh's Dr. Anne Mari Yali, women who are optimists are more likely to *believe* they have control over their pregnancy, so they are less stressed. With less stress, she says, you can have a better pregnancy outcome—so, in a sense, believing that you *can* impact your pregnancy really *gives you* that control. Studies presented at the 1999 annual meeting of the Society of Behavioral Medicine validated this power of positive thinking. Here it was reported that less optimistic women had a high degree of early delivery and low-birthweight babies compared to women who were positive thinkers. The finding remained true even after doctors controlled for factors that could affect results, such as smoking, diet, and diabetes. Echoing these findings—a Danish study revealed that even major life stressors had little impact on pregnancy if the problems were not identified as being personally stressful to the mother.

TIME OUT FOR STRESS REDUCTION

In addition to maintaining a positive outlook, experts say that it's also important to make time in your life for stress-busting activities—things that you enjoy doing *and* that can help you relax. Doing so can be doubly important when you are experiencing extreme stress. Taking a brief time-out may even eliminate some of the effects of stress hormones. So, read a book, watch a soap opera, have a cup of herbal tea, take a nap—whatever breaks the tension for you can reduce stress and promote the health of your pregnancy.

You also can take some of the sting out of even extremely stressful situations if you take a few small steps to modify what you can about your circumstances. Sometimes even taking a small positive step in the midst of a tragedy can make you feel more in control and less helpless. Ultimately, that can help you to feel less stressed. So can stress-reducing activities, such as meditation, yoga, even listening to music or having a pregnancy massage. "There is ample evidence that these activities can affect physical responses to anxiety, such as lowering heart rate and stress hormone levels," reports New York University reproductive psychiatrist Dr. Shari Lusskin.

Stress and Your Lifestyle:
What You Need to Know

As you probably already know, cigarettes, alcohol, and recreational drugs can have some pretty devastating effects on your pregnancy, increasing health risks for both you and your baby. But what you might not realize is how their negative effects can be intensified when stress enters the equation. In at least one study, doctors found that the threat of stress-related miscarriage increased up to threefold in women who smoked.

Unfortunately, when we are stressed, studies show we often turn to risky behaviors. In an effort to cope, we may drink or smoke more, and sometimes even turn to drugs or compulsive eating as a way to alleviate fears and anxieties. That's why it's doubly important to be strong and not give in to unhealthy cravings or urges simply because you feel stressed.

Real Life

STRESS, PREGNANCY, AND MEMORY

Q: Ever since I've been pregnant, I find my memory is not what it used to be—I'm even forgetting simple things, like where I put my car keys or where I parked my car! My husband says it's all stress—and I do admit I am a bit nervous about the baby. But is there any other reason I could be losing my memory? I'm worried that maybe something else is wrong.

A: Yes, it's true, stress can affect our memory—and the more you worry about not being able to remember, the more stressed you will feel, and the less you will remember! That said, studies show that short-term memory loss can also occur in pregnant women who *aren't* stressed. In research appearing in the *Journal of Reproductive Medicine* in early 2002, doctors reported that a drop in blood levels of three important brain chemicals linked to memory occur during pregnancy—the neurotransmitters serotonin, dopamine, and epinephrine. Further, these drops coincide with the time frame of the most dramatic memory losses reported by women—late in the first trimester and continuing into the second trimester. While researchers say they don't know what causes these brain chemicals to falter or why some women are affected more than others, studies do show that memory usually increases again in the third trimester. Moreover, doctors say it often rebounds fully shortly after birth. However, if you are breast-feeding, regaining your full capacity to remember may take a bit longer. Swedish studies conducted as far back as 1990 found that increased levels of the biochemical oxytocin (which soars during breast-feeding) may temporarily affect memory for up to twelve months after your baby is born, though you are likely to see gradual improvement over that time frame.

Remember, these substances can ultimately make your stress worse and, in the process, do some real harm to both you and your baby.

Whenever possible, work off stressful feelings with more health-giving activities such as exercise: Go for a walk when the stress builds, or spend some time on an exercise bike. If eating helps break the stress, opt for healthy snacks, such as high-protein, high-calcium, low-fat treats, like frozen yogurt. These can provide some "food comfort" while still giving you some of the nutrients you need for a healthy pregnancy.

Coping with Stress Naturally: What You Can Do

While it's true that your sense of smell is exaggerated during pregnancy—and for many women nearly all scents can be taboo—for some, fragrances can become a saving grace, helping you beat even the most stressful times. The reason is aromatherapy, the gentle art—some say science—of blending essential aromatic oils in a way that can significantly impact your body, mind, and spirit. Indeed, research shows that when the nose detects the aroma of an essential oil, nerve impulses send a message to an area of the brain known as the limbic system. Here we find cells that not only control memory and emotion, but also the pituitary gland, which is the "master control" of all hormone production, including those biochemicals influenced by stress. Ultimately, aromatherapy can be a powerful agent, helping you not only to relax, but also to control certain stress-related pregnancy complaints such as insomnia or fatigue.

Although a wide variety of fragrances can help reduce stress, not every scent used in aromatherapy is safe to use during pregnancy. This is because some can have a stimulating effect on the uterus that may induce contractions. That means you can't automatically substitute essential oils in a pregnancy formulation or use certain oils simply because you like the way they smell.

Those oils considered generally safe to use during pregnancy include gentle scents such as chamomile, citrus (lemon, orange, bergamot, mandarin, and neroli), frankincense, geranium, lavender, and sandalwood. Some experts also recommend cypress, patchouli, tea tree oil, and ylang-ylang, plus clary sage and rosemary if used during the third trimester only. Jasmine, peppermint, and rose are also okay anytime after the sixteenth week of pregnancy. If the scents of these essential oils don't appeal to you, then consult with a professional aromatherapist about what you can safely use. Often your favorite essential oil can be made "safer" for use during pregnancy, by either diluting the dosage or combining it with certain other oils.

Never use an essential oil directly on your skin. Doing so can net you a nasty burn or a skin inflammation. Always dilute essential oils in a carrier oil such as sweet almond, jojoba, or olive oil.

To help you start putting aromatherapy to work in your life, here are a few "classic" recipes recommended for stress reduction during pregnancy. However, because every pregnancy is unique and different, it's important that you **check with your obstetrician before using any essential oil preparation.**

THE AROMATHERAPY BATH

Into a tub of warm water you can add one of the following aromatherapy formulas:

For relaxation: Combine 2 drops each of neroli, lavender, and lemon oil with 6 teaspoons of sweet almond oil, olive oil, or jojoba oil.

For nervous tension: Combine 2 drops each of lavender, geranium, and rose oil with 6 teaspoons of apricot kernel or sweet almond oil.

FOR NERVOUS ANXIETY

Into a 10 milliliter bottle, place 3 drops of lavender and 1 drop of neroli oil. Add vegetable oil to fill and mix well. Put several drops in hands and inhale; massage temples, neck, and forehead.

FOR GENERAL RELAXATION

Into a 10 milliliter bottle add 2 drops of bergamot, 2 drops of orange, and 1 drop of neroli oils. Add vegetable oil to fill. Rub on hands and inhale. (Option: After the second trimester, you can exchange rose for neroli oil, if you prefer this scent.)

If whipping up creams, lotions, and bath oils is not exactly your idea of pampering care, you can simply place a few drops of these essential oil recipes into a bowl of water, allowing the scent to waft into your environment. Using a heated diffuser, usually powered by a candle or lightbulb, can help spread the aroma quicker and make it much stronger.

The Pregnancy Massage:
The Ultimate Stress Reducer

For many women, the ultimate way to reduce stress and really relax is a full-body massage. During pregnancy this can be even more important, as it not only soothes your jangled nerves, but also helps relax tired, aching muscles and reduces swelling in hands and feet. Studies also show that the simple act of touch can dramatically reduce the production of stress hormones, lessen anxiety, and improve sleep. In studies conducted at Touch Research Institute at the University of Miami, just twenty minutes of massage twice weekly for five weeks improved the moods and sleep patterns of pregnant women, while reducing anxiety and back pain. Additionally, doctors were able to measure a significant difference in the level of stress hormones secreted in the urine of pregnant women who received regular massage. In 1999 a similar study published in the *Journal of Psychosomatic Obstetrics and Gynecology* reported pregnant women who underwent massage therapy experienced less anxiety, a decrease in stress hormones, and fewer obstetrical and postnatal complications. But Mom isn't the only one to benefit from massage—baby does too! The journal also reported lower rates of premature birth among mothers who were massaged, while the Touch Research Institute study reported that infants of mothers who underwent massage had fewer postnatal complications.

While having a professional massage was once considered a luxury few could afford, today massage therapists are far less expensive than ever before. And, with the health benefits of massage now so clearly defined, some insurance companies may even pay some or all of the costs, depending on your policy. But even if you have to pay on your own, many hospitals now offer massage therapy options right along with childbirth classes at a nominal fee.

When choosing a therapist on your own, make certain to seek out someone who is trained *and certified* in pregnancy massage. This is imperative if you are going to have a safe and beneficial experience. To find a certified massage therapist in your area or to check on the credentials of one you've found on your own, contact the National Association of Pregnancy Massage Therapists (NAPMT) at 888-451-4945 or e-mail them at NAPMT@Texas.net.

In addition, registered massage therapist and certified pregnancy expert Kelly Lott offers these important tips for making your pregnancy massage experience safer and healthier:

- Never get a massage during your first trimester. While there is no clear-cut evidence to show massage at this time is harmful, experts say there is a potential to increase the risk of miscarriage. Instead wait until your second or third trimester, when the benefits will be even greater.

- You should never experience pain during a massage. If you do, tell your therapist to stop immediately.

- Never lie on your back for a massage after the twentieth week of pregnancy; doing so could compromise blood flow to your uterus and harm your baby.

- Your therapist should never massage open sores, areas where you have a rash, over raised or distended varicose veins, or around or near any local site of infection.

- Avoid pressure between the ankle bone and the heel, as well as to the webbing between toes. Many massage therapists and reflexologists caution that these points on the body directly correlate to the uterus and vagina, and heavy pressure, particularly in the third trimester, could induce premature labor.

- Avoid massage on the abdomen; it could start baby kicking, and there goes Mom's relaxation time!

While your pregnancy massage can be as short as ten minutes or as long as sixty minutes, it's not a good idea to go beyond that time limit, no matter how great it feels. During your second trimester, you can have a massage once a week; during your third trimester, you can increase massages to twice weekly or more, if needed.

Unless you are having an aromatherapy massage, experts say an unscented lotion is best. If your therapist is using a scented lotion or oil, make certain to smell it before it's applied to your body—even if it's something you've used before. Remember, your sense of smell changes during pregnancy, and the scents you loved before conception may not smell so great to you now.

Important Warning about Pregnancy Massage: As beneficial as a pregnancy massage can be, it's not right for every pregnant woman. For this reason, before you schedule a massage, check with your doctor. In fact, this may even be necessary, since some professional massage therapists require a doctor's note stating that a pregnancy massage is okay.

Issues that might suggest a massage is not for you include heart disease, hypertension, diabetes, asthma, a previous pregnancy with complications, or if you are carrying twins, triplets, or quadruplets. Also avoid pregnancy massage if: you have any unexplained pain in your abdomen; you are in danger of losing your pregnancy; you are experiencing fever, nausea, or vomiting; you have an unusually heavy discharge of water or blood; or your doctor has diagnosed you with preeclampsia or toxemia, a form of pregnancy-related high blood pressure.

Partner Massage: What You Need to Know

For many women, the ultimate stress-busting pregnancy massage is one from a loving partner. And, in fact, childbirth experts agree that when Dad massages Mom, both become more relaxed and more involved with the pregnancy. Sometimes parental bonding with baby can begin even before birth—something that studies show can help Mom feel a lot more relaxed.

If either you or your partner feels a little hesitant to attempt a pregnancy massage, many hospitals and birthing centers offer classes, where your first rubdown is conducted under the watchful eye of a certified instructor. If, however, you both feel comfortable enough to give it a go on your own, nurse/midwife Margaret Fawcett offers the following simple massage techniques for you to try.

Important: Regardless of who is doing your massage, make certain they pay attention to the safety tips highlighted earlier in this chapter.

THE LOVING PARTNER BACK MASSAGE

Perhaps the most difficult part of getting a home massage is finding a comfortable position and a spot for your pampering pleasure to take place. This is particularly true for back massage, since lying on your stomach is a definite no, particularly during the later months of pregnancy. What can work: straddling a chair, with the back facing your front. This works especially well if you place the chair in front of a table and then stack one or two pillows over the back, allowing them to spill out on to the tabletop. By doing so you will be able to lean forward during the massage.

An alternate position: Kneel on the floor with your knees apart and your heels tucked under your buttocks. A stack of pillows placed in front will allow you to lean forward, while a pillow under your belly and another over your heels and under your buttocks will help cushion and support your body.

Starting Your Massage: Before starting your massage, your partner should always warm the oil or lotion by pouring a small amount into his hands and rubbing them together. This is an important step, since anything cold causes muscles to tense, which will cause you to feel stressed. Any high-quality commercial massage oil can work, or make your own by combining a few drops of a relaxing essential oil such as lavender or chamomile with sweet almond or jojoba oil. (See recipes below.) Or you can simply use any body lotion you like.

To begin: Your partner should place his hands on your lower back just below the waistline and slowly begin sliding up your back on either side of your spine. **He must never massage directly on your backbone or over your spinal column.** As he reaches the shoulders, he should slowly move his hands across your upper back, then down the opposite side of your spine, to the starting point. This up-and-down motion should continue for at least several minutes, until the muscles of your back start to warm and relax. Once you feel this sense of muscle relaxation, your partner can begin applying gentle pressure to any area of your back where you are feeling pain, using the heel of the hand or the pads of the fingers, bearing down slightly and continuing to move in a circular

Mother *Nature* Knows Best

MAKE YOUR OWN
ULTRA-RELAXING MASSAGE OIL

For a quick, fragrant, and relaxing massage oil, add 1 teaspoon of carrier oil (such as sweet almond, apricot kernel, vitamin E, or olive oil) for
every drop of essential oil. Use no more than 3 drops for any one massage. If you are sensitive to smells, single oils work best—such as lavender, chamomile, or citrus. If you already have a blend you like for your
bath, use that, as long as you never use more than 1 drop of fragrance
per teaspoon of carrier oil. Always patch test an essential oil mixture on
the inside of your elbow for twenty-four hours before using it as a massage or bath oil.

motion. The operative word here is "gentle." The point of massage is to
relax and soothe muscles, so a rubdown should *never* hurt. If it does, your
partner is pressing too hard, so let him know you are experiencing discomfort. Your massage finishes with a repeat of the up-and-down motion
that started your back rub for several more minutes. Then wrap your
body in a soft blanket or beach towel to keep muscles warm, and remain
in your massage position for five to ten minutes.

Coping with Major Stress: What You Can Do

Whether your stress is related to a community or national event or the result of a deeply personal experience, sometimes you are going to need
something more than just a back rub or hot bath to reduce anxious feelings. Experts from the American College of Obstetricians and Gynecologists offer the following tips to help you deal with the stressors in your
life, and keep your pregnancy on track.

> • *Keep a pregnancy diary—and make it a point to enter at least one
> thing you do for yourself every day.* This will remind you of the im-

portance of taking care of and, yes, even pampering yourself during your pregnancy.

- *Talk about your feelings.* Whether you are stressed, fearful, physically ill, worried about your health or that of your baby, or even have doubts about motherhood itself, talk to your doctor, your partner, your family or friends, and, if necessary, a counselor who can give you objective advice.

- *Turn off the TV news.* Instead watch a comedy or educational show or hunt for bargains on a television shopping network. According to experts, watching frightening or upsetting news stories, particularly seeing them repeated over and over, can increase stress levels significantly. Taking your mind off stressful events by, say, shopping on TV can go a long way in relieving your stress.

- *Exercise moderately and regularly.* Not only can exercise make you feel stronger and more in control of your body and your pregnancy, brain chemicals produced during exercise can make you feel calmer.

- *Learn labor relaxation exercises, and do them every day—they're great stress-busters!* Many of these routines, particularly the breathing exercises, focus on relaxation. Not only will doing them daily help you be ultra-prepared for labor; the exercises themselves can help calm you down and alleviate stress *during* pregnancy.

- *Don't take over-the-counter or herbal stress medicines in an attempt to calm down or get to sleep.* Some can be dangerous during pregnancy or may make you feel worse. Instead, talk to your doctor about what prescription medications may be okay for short-term stress control.

- *If feelings of stress, fear, or anxiety seem overwhelming, consider talking to a pregnancy counselor—a mental health professional trained to deal with the emotional side of pregnancy.* Most often, your doctor can recommend someone—or call the obstetrics department of your local hospital and ask for a reference.

• *Finally, don't get stressed over feeling stressed!* If something upsetting does occur during your pregnancy, try not to panic. Maintain a positive attitude and make time to talk to your doctor about whatever is causing you fear and worry.

To Sleep, Perchance to Dream

Among the best ways to reduce stress in your life is to make certain you get the proper amount of sleep. One reason is that sleep deprivation not only causes stress, it can exacerbate the effects of whatever kinds of problems are present in your life.

But as important as getting a good night's sleep can be, it's not always so easy to accomplish. According to the National Sleep Foundation, 78 percent of women surveyed experienced more sleep problems during pregnancy than at any other time in their life—and experts point to the hormone progesterone as the main cause. While surges of this hormone occurring early in pregnancy are often responsible for making you feel fatigued, ironically, these same surges can keep you from falling asleep at night.

A six-year study conducted by Kathryn Lee, professor of nursing at the University of California–San Francisco, found that even when you do finally get to sleep, pregnancy hormones can cause you to spend more time in the REM (rapid eye movement) stage, rather than progressing to the deeper stages necessary to fight fatigue. Her study, published in the journal *Obstetrics and Gynecology* in early 2000, also showed that both the number of hours you sleep during pregnancy and the depth of your sleep can drop dramatically starting as early as the eleventh week after conception. Not coincidentally, most women also find that they dream a lot more during pregnancy—with strong, vivid, and even frightening images that can also interfere with sleep. (See "I Dreamed I Ate My Baby!" later in this chapter.)

But hormones aren't the only things keeping you awake at night. For many women the physical symptoms of pregnancy cause the most problems—particularly frequent nighttime trips to the bathroom. Because blood volume expands to almost double during pregnancy, your kidneys are working overtime to cleanse that blood—and in the process making

twice the amount of urine. This, coupled with the pressure of your growing baby on your bladder, means you have to urinate more often, particularly at night.

Other pregnancy-related complaints that may be interfering with
your sleep include gastrointestinal upsets, nausea, heartburn, pain from
hemorrhoids, and restless leg syndrome (RLS)—temporary but annoying
sensations in your limbs that can keep you awake all night. While some
of these problems will improve beginning as early as your second
trimester—when baby moves away from your bladder and your hormones
calm down—come trimester three, baby moves again *and* your belly and
breasts really enlarge, so you can expect some sleep problems to recur.

Seven Super Solutions for
Getting the Sleep You Need

While getting enough sleep can be a challenge during pregnancy, it's not
impossible. In fact, when it comes to sleep solutions, the key, say doctors,
is to "think outside the box." Look below the surface to identify *your* particular sleep problems, then seek out some creative ways around the factors keeping you awake at night. To get you started thinking in the right
direction, the National Sleep Foundation and experts from the American
College of Obstetricians and Gynecologists offer these solutions to help
you get the sleep you and your baby need.

SOLUTION #1: LEARN TO POWER NAP

Among the biggest misconceptions about pregnancy sleep is that it must
take place at night, in bed, in order to count. Nothing could be further
from the truth. Sleep is sleep—and when you are pregnant, you should
grab it every chance you get. That means taking advantage of those sleepy,
lazy feelings that hit midafternoon by catching a nap. The National Sleep
Foundation reports that more than half of all pregnant women say they
napped on weekday afternoons, while more than 60 percent said they
napped on weekends. And, remember that your nap doesn't have to be
very long to be effective. A new Australian study conducted at the School
of Psychology Sleep Laboratory in Adelaide showed that ten minutes of

sleep can be extremely effective when it comes to boosting performance for up to three hours afterward.

SOLUTION #2: LIMIT FLUID INTAKE AND WATCH BEDTIME SNACKS

If frequent trips to the bathroom are disrupting your sleep, one solution is to avoid drinking anything beginning two hours before bedtime. While maintaining adequate fluid intake is vital during pregnancy, it can be taxing to your kidneys. By drinking most of your fluids during the daytime hours, your kidneys—along with your psyche—can rest better at night.

If you haven't already banished caffeine from your diet, doing so now can help. Not only will caffeine keep you awake, it also promotes urination. If you can't quit, then limit caffeine consumption—including tea and hot chocolate—before bedtime. According to the National Sleep Foundation, you should also limit heavy, spicy, or acidic foods close to bedtime, particularly if heartburn or indigestion keeps you awake. If you do need a bedtime snack, try crackers or any high-carbohydrate food, which can fill you up and help you feel more sleepy.

If headaches, bad dreams, or night sweats are your main sleeptime problem, eating a high-protein snack before bedtime—such as a hard-boiled egg or some cottage cheese—may help you sleep more soundly. If heartburn persists and is keeping you awake, try sleeping with your head and chest elevated. This can help keep acid in your stomach from moving up into your chest, where it causes the burn.

SOLUTION #3: GET COMFY!

While it may seem that the words "comfort" and "pregnancy" don't belong in the same sentence, this doesn't have to be the case. Small changes in sleeping habits and routines *can* make a huge difference.

First and foremost, experts say don't sleep on your back. Doing so is likely to cause excess strain on your spine and intestines, and it can also constrict the vein that transports blood from your lower body to your heart. This, in turn, can impede circulation and cause impaired breathing—both of which are not only uncomfortable for you but dangerous for your baby. The best position for both of you is when you lie on your left side.

As your tummy begins to grow, experiment with pillow support, using them in various ways to prop up your back and your belly. Slipping still another pillow between your knees can help take pressure off your spine and increase your comfort level. While some women just adore pillows specifically designed for pregnancy, including the "wedge," you can get somewhat the same results by manipulating bed or couch pillows you already have. If getting comfortable is really a problem, you might want to invest in a contoured foam mattress topper, which works well to take stress off pressure points like hipbones, elbows, and knees.

SOLUTION #4: DRESS FOR SLEEP SUCCESS

Wearing comfy clothes while you sleep is a given—and the looser they are during pregnancy, the better you will feel. But in addition to feeling comfortable, your pregnant body also needs support, and wearing some undergarments while you sleep can be a big plus in establishing a new level of comfort.

Among the two most important items are a sleeping bra and a pregnancy support belt. A sleeping bra can help keep breasts from hurting and keep them slightly lifted off your tummy, which can make breathing easier. If you don't want to spend the money for a sleeping bra, you can wear your regular daytime bra, but do loosen the straps and close it using the first row of hooks only.

A belly belt will support your abdomen, asleep and awake, as well as relieve back pain and take some pressure off your bladder. The belts, which wrap around the waist and then utilize a strap that goes under the tummy, are made of elastic, so they move when you move while still offering support. (See Chapter 4.)

SOLUTION #5: BEDTIME EXERCISE AND GENTLE MASSAGE

While a strenuous workout close to bedtime can keep you awake, gentle exercises—particularly stretching—can relax your body and ease minor

Mother *Nature* Knows Best

SLEEP SOLUTIONS FROM YOUR KITCHEN AND GARDEN

To help you get a better night's sleep, try the following:

✓ **Warm Milk and Cookies.** The milk contains an amino acid known as tryptophan, which raises levels of the brain chemical serotonin—nature's own powerful relaxant. The cookies are carbohydrates, which can also help make you sleepy. There's also something to be said for the relaxing effects of comfort goodies like cookies and milk. One caveat: If you suffer from RLS—restless leg syndrome—skip the cookies. A high-carb snack could encourage this problem and may keep you from sleeping.

✓ **Chamomile Tea.** This relaxing beverage not only helps your body to feel warm and calm all over, it has particularly good effects on your digestive system, helping to ease gastric complaints and heartburn associated with pregnancy. Chamomile is also one of the few herbs deemed safe by the Food and Drug Administration for ingestion during pregnancy.

   Important note: If you have ragweed allergy or hayfever, you might be be allergic to chamomile. To test yourself, hold tea in your mouth for thirty seconds and spit out; if your tongue or cheeks feel itchy or strange, it could be an allergy.

✓ **Lavender Pillows.** Lavender is one of the most relaxing herbs you can find. Dusting pillows with lavender powder or sprinkling some lavender herb inside your pillowcase can do wonders for helping you relax and gently fall asleep. You can even find a lavender-scented linen spray for sheets and pillowcases. Do, however, choose only products scented with English or French lavender. The Spanish variety can be stimulating and may keep you up all night.

aches and pains, helping you to fall asleep faster. Experts say to do your stretches about two hours before bedtime and, when you can, follow with a ten- or twenty-minute soak in a warm bath. If possible, ask your partner for a back massage just prior to bedtime, which can relax muscles and help you fall asleep.

SOLUTION #6: IMAGINE THE PATH TO DREAMLAND

If your sleep problems are more the result of fears and worries than actual physical discomforts, taking steps to transport your mind to a more relaxed place can carry you off to dreamland in the process. Among the easiest ways to accomplish both is through the use of guided imagery—a way of vividly imagining you are in any pleasant situation you choose.

"You simply imagine a peaceful scene—a place that is comforting and consoling—a kind of oasis where you can imagine yourself free of problems, particularly pain," says Dr. Mehmet Oz, director of the Cardiovascular Institute at Columbia Presbyterian Medical Center and one of a growing number of physicians who have studied the effects of guided imagery. When the mind "digests" these peaceful images, the effects are felt in the body—and therein lie the restorative properties. Many hospitals around the nation are now instituting guided imagery programs as part of routine patient care. When combined with a deep and rhythmic breathing exercise just prior to bedtime, guided imagery can help you overcome pregnancy worries and help you get a deeper, more restful night's sleep.

To learn more about how to use guided imagery during pregnancy and obtain a free program, check out www.eupsychia.com/perspectives/imagery.html. For a free sample of several professional guided imagery tapes and CDs that use both music and voice to help you relax, visit www.serenitymusic.com/guided.html.

SOLUTION #7: HAVE SEX AS OFTEN AS YOU CAN

While it may not be the first thing on your mind, sex *can* be a great way to relax your body—not to mention distract your mind—and help you fall asleep naturally. Though initially stimulating, once orgasm occurs, a series

Real Life

SNORING LIKE A WILD BEAST

Q: I know I never had a snoring problem, and now, suddenly, my husband tells me I snore like a wild beast every night. I didn't believe him at first, but then one night he taped me snoring—and it was horrifying! I sounded like a wild bear in heat! Is this anything to be concerned about?

A: I'm a little concerned that you actually know what a wild bear in heat *sounds* like, but other than that, there is probably little cause for real concern! According to the National Sleep Foundation, up to 30 percent of all pregnant women snore—even if they never did so before. The problem is often caused by increased swelling in the nasal passages that sometimes occurs during pregnancy, partially blocking your airways. For most women this is harmless and temporary. That said, one study published in January 2000 in the journal *Chest* found that women who began snoring during pregnancy were at increased risk for high blood pressure, preeclampsia, abnormal accumulation of fluid in the tissues, and more weight gain. The women also gave birth to smaller babies, who each scored lower on postbirth physical tests. According to the study author, Dr. Karl A. Franklin, the consequences of compromising your ability to breathe during sleep may affect your baby, supporting a previously suggested relationship between sleep apnea and intrauterine growth retardation. In sleep apnea, the blockage of air becomes so severe you actually stop breathing for a few seconds numerous times during the night. This lack of oxygen not only encourages loud snoring, but also disrupts sleep and affects the oxygen supply to your baby. While sleep and pregnancy experts are waiting for more studies before they accept these findings, to be on the safe side, check with your doctor about your snoring, particularly if, despite sleeping all night, you are still exhausted the next day. Extreme fatigue coupled with very loud snoring is sometimes a sign of sleep apnea.

of biochemical events take your body into a deep state of relaxation that ultimately can make falling asleep easier. Another bonus: For many women, their sexy new pregnancy body chemistry can make arousal more potent and climax easier to obtain!

While most of the time intercourse as well as orgasm are okay—usually right up until the very last stage of your third trimester—do check with your doctor about how late in your pregnancy is safe for you. In rare instances—when you are in danger of premature labor, for example—you may need to take some extra precautions in regard to sexual activity. (See Chapter 8 for more information on sex during pregnancy.)

Calming Your Pregnancy Fears: What Every Woman Can Do

Along with the joy you are experiencing about being pregnant, don't be surprised if you are also facing down some fears, particularly if this is your first baby. For most women, these fears will be centered around the health of their pregnancy and the birth of a healthy baby. For a few, however, this may also be a time of extreme introspection. You may find yourself examining your life and even your reason for wanting a baby—perhaps for the very first time. You may even wonder whether parenthood is really right for you, as you question whether it's the best time to have a baby, or if your career or your relationship with your partner may suffer or change. While on one hand you may feel happy to be pregnant, on the other, you may at times find yourself acting like a spoiled little child, angry and resentful that you can't participate in some of the activities or opportunities that you could before getting pregnant.

While the vast majority of women *won't* feel this way, reproductive psychiatrist Dr. Shari Lusskin advises that those who do may have a strained relationship with their own mother—one that causes a variety of mother-child conflicts and fears to come to the forefront during pregnancy, sometimes creating a great deal of stress for the mother-to-be. In this respect, pregnancy can be a good time to tackle those hidden conflicts and bring them into the open, allowing you to move into motherhood a healthier and happier person. Certainly, some women report find-

Real Life

I DREAMED I ATE MY BABY

Q: I don't have trouble getting to sleep, but when I do, I have these horrendous nightmares—scary, vivid dreams about things like biting off my baby's head. The dreams are so scary and so real I often can't go back to sleep—and when I do, I sometimes go right back into the same horrible dream. Now it's so bad, I don't even want to sleep at all; it's like I become some kind of monster the minute my eyes are closed. I'm too frightened to tell my doctor—he'll think I'm totally crazy. Am I?

A: Relax! You're not crazy or a monster. And chances are excellent you won't do anything more than nibble your baby's ear and smother her in kisses once she's born. Thanks to pregnancy hormones, dramatic, vivid, and even scary dreams are *common* during pregnancy—and most women have at least a few, if not many, beginning soon after conception. Pregnancy dream therapists Sindy Greenberg and Elyse Kroll say our dreams represent a compilation of our mostly old, unsettled unconscious conflicts, along with our newer, more recent conscious conflicts—our thoughts about what's going on in our life at the moment. "By allowing ourselves to review our conflicts while we sleep, we're attempting to work through and cope with the issues that are troubling us," they write in their book *Dreaming for Two*. During pregnancy, they say, our dreams—even the seemingly scary ones—can actually help ease us into motherhood.

As to your nightmare about biting off your baby's head, experts say it could be a fear of not being able to care for your baby once she is born, or concerns that you may not be a good or protective mother—fears that are common during pregnancy. Think about what's really bothering or scaring you, and then make a list of creative solutions or reasons why you shouldn't be worried. Read the list right before going to sleep, and you might find your dreams take on a less ominous tone.

ing solace in simply knowing that others share their concerns; books of essays like *Child of Mine* can help you to explore your feelings. In many instances, however, more may be accomplished via one of the newer forms of obstetrical care—a speciality known as reproductive psychiatry. These doctors specialize in helping women with emotional conflicts that either stem from, or are made worse by, becoming pregnant. Don't be shy about asking your doctor for a referral to a counselor who can help you work through your conflicted feelings so that you emerge from your pregnancy not only a strong and well-adjusted mother, but a stronger and happier person overall.

For most of you, however, pregnancy fears and worries will be centered not on yourself but on your baby and the anxieties connected to giving birth. As you enter your second trimester and hormones calm down, you will most likely begin to feel better. However, as you enter your third trimester, Dr. Lusskin says, don't be surprised if fears reappear as labor and childbirth grow closer.

The important thing to remember, however, is that in most instances, most of your fears *will never come to pass.* Moreover, because they are not anxieties that stem from some deep-seated conflicts but simply from a fear of the unknown, there are things you can do to help keep your stressful feelings under control.

With the advice of childbirth experts from the University of Iowa's department of nursing and Dr. Lusskin, here are some strategies for combating the most common fears and concerns that develop during pregnancy.

Top Eight Pregnancy Fears and How to Conquer Them

#1: FEAR THAT SOMETHING IS WRONG WITH YOUR BABY

What to Do: First realize that the overwhelming percentage of babies born today are perfect, healthy babies, and the odds are overwhelmingly in your favor. If you still have concerns, talk to your doctor about whether you might benefit from an ultrasound, amniocentesis, or alpha fetal protein test; any or all can reassure you that your baby is just fine.

#2: FEAR OF PAIN DURING CHILDBIRTH

What to Do: Once again your doctor can help, by providing you with as much information as possible about safe, new pain relief options—and there are plenty of them. You should also learn a little about cesarean section deliveries so, in the event that this becomes necessary, you'll feel strong and prepared, and not overwhelmed and confused.

#3: FEAR OF NOT BEING A GOOD MOTHER

What to Do: Recognize that this is a very normal concern and may be even more prevalent if you have a strained relationship with your own mother. Realize that much of what it takes to be a mother will come quite naturally to you once baby is born, even if you think you'll be all thumbs now. Reading some books on child development can help, as can talking to friends or family members with young children, so you know what to expect in the weeks and months that follow childbirth.

#4: FEAR OF MISCARRIAGE

What to Do: Studies published as early as 1980 cited this fear as among the most common in pregnant women of all ages, first-time mothers as well as experienced moms. Most prevalent during the first trimester, you can overcome at least some of this anxiety by eating nutritiously and exercising, both of which can make you feel confident and strong—and that, in turn, can alleviate some of your fears. In addition, recognize that guilt is a common precipitator of fear, so, if you make every effort to live a healthy lifestyle during pregnancy—no smoking, drinking, or drug use—then you may alleviate guilt, which in turn can alleviate those fears.

#5: FEAR OF HAVING YOUR BABY IN THE BACK OF A TAXI (ON A TRAIN, IN THE EMPLOYEE CAFETERIA, IN THE LADIES' ROOM, ETC.)

What to Do: While we've all heard the stories of babies being born in unusual places, remember that what makes them headlines is that these events happen so *infrequently.* For most women—particularly those having their first child—labor will be a very identifiable event, and not something likely to sneak up on you in the middle of a board meeting or at the grocery store. What can help is educating yourself on the stages of labor—what comes first and how to recognize the signs—and then having a plan of action in mind for when the event begins. Know whom you are going to call, how you will get to the hospital, and how you will reach your partner, and have backups for everyone on your list.

#6: FEAR OF EMBARRASSING YOURSELF DURING DELIVERY

What to Do: First, remember that no matter what you can possibly imagine might happen, your doctors and the labor and delivery staff have *seen it all.* There likely isn't anything you might do, or any reaction you might have, that's going to surprise anyone.

That said, you should also stop listening to all those delivery-day horror stories that friends, neighbors, and relatives just can't seem to stop telling you since you became pregnant. In reality, the likelihood of something really embarrassing happening to you is *very small.*

#7: FEAR OF LOSS OF INTIMACY/SEX/LIFESTYLE WITH YOUR PARTNER

What to Do: Talk to your partner and share your feelings, particularly if you feel insecure or unattractive with your pregnant body. You might be surprised to learn just how desirable you are, even as you are about to give birth!

It's also important to realize that, in the days and weeks that follow childbirth, your changing hormones along with physical problems related to the birth itself may cause you to feel ambiguous or even turned off to any kind of sex or intimate contact. Again, the solution here is to talk to your partner and make certain he understands that the way you are feeling is a natural part of pregnancy and only temporary. (See Chapter 8.) In terms of fears over resuming a satisfying sex life after pregnancy—remember the wonders of the Kegel exercise! If you continue the Kegels you started during pregnancy (see Chapter 5), you can keep your V zone toned, healthy, and ready for intimacy whenever you are.

#8: FEAR OF FAT, NOT BEING ATTRACTIVE, LOSING YOUR FIGURE

What to Do: When compared to fears about miscarriage or labor and delivery, a fear of figure flaws may seem very shallow to many women. Still, don't be surprised if this *does* become one of your concerns, particularly during your third trimester. As you begin to approach your due date, you may feel somewhat overwhelmed by your size and by your ability to lose the extra weight after baby is born. This might be particularly true if you struggled to control your weight before pregnancy. To overcome this fear—or even to prevent it from developing—take good dietary control of your pregnancy right from the start. If you eat a healthy, nutritious diet, getting extra calories from lots of fresh fruits and vegetables and lean meat and poultry (and not from cookies, cake, and ice cream), studies show your weight will be easier to lose afterward. Studies also show that if you exercise during your pregnancy, you'll be less likely to gain excess weight and more likely to lose it after baby is born.

Your Pregnancy State of Mind: A Final Word

Certainly, no one can predict exactly how your pregnancy will go or guarantee that your fears will never be realized. Still, it's extremely important to understand that most pregnancies turn out just fine. The majority of babies *are* born healthy and perfect, and, despite those delivery-day horror stories, most moms have far fewer complications than they feared or imagined.

It's also important that you acknowledge the idea that, yes, having a baby *is* going to cause some profound changes in your life and your lifestyle. In fact, it is guaranteed that things will never be quite the same again! However, with a little bit of time and a few adjustments now and again, you and your partner will mostly likely find that your new "family life" is one filled with excitement and great joy.

Also remember that most women experience some stress, anxiety, and even fear during pregnancy—and that this is quite common. But if these feelings, or your levels of stress, become significant—if you can't think or do anything except focus on your negative feelings—make certain you talk to your doctor. The important thing is that you don't try to go it alone.

"Pregnancy is a time when, for some women, childhood fears and anxieties come to the forefront—so it can be an opportunity to confront and work out issues that have been tucked away for a very long time," says Dr. Lusskin. In many instances, all you may need are some reassuring words to calm your stress and quell your fears.

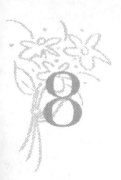

Sex and Pregnancy

Answers to Your Most Intimate Questions

You're bloated, nauseous, and more tired than you've ever been in your life, and sex is so far out of the picture it's not even on your radar screen.

Or you're feeling steamy, hot, sensuous, and wanting your partner more than you ever thought you could.

Sound like two different women? It could be. But don't be surprised if these kinds of dramatic sexual mood swings are part of a single pregnancy: yours. While most women are fairly well acquainted with their sexual appetite prior to conceiving, once pregnancy happens, everything you thought you knew about your need or desire for sex may suddenly change. What's more, the minute you think you've figured it all out, you enter a new trimester and things can change once again.

Complicating matters a bit further, either you or your partner may be harboring some secret (or not so secret) fears and worries about engaging in sex during pregnancy. Even couples who want and need intimate contact during this time may find themselves abstaining, simply because they are fearful that something they do may harm their baby.

The good news is that sex and pregnancy are a healthy combination, one that can benefit you and, when it comes time for labor and delivery, even your baby. Physically and emotionally, the fact is, sex can help keep you and your partner close, keep your pelvic floor muscles toned for delivery, and help with body issues generated by your pregnancy size, allowing you to feel more sexy and desirable. And, in most instances, it's safe! In fact, with just a little bit of understanding about what is happening to your body—and why—plus a few key facts about sex during pregnancy, you can be well on your way to a healthy and happy intimate relationship that lasts all nine months and beyond. And while it may seem hard to imagine right now, for some of you pregnancy may turn out to be one of the most sexually exciting times of your life!

Pregnancy and Sexual Desire: What You Need to Know

Perhaps the most important thing you can learn about sexual desire and pregnancy is that no two days are going to be alike. Much like the time before you conceived, some days you will feel like having sex, other days you won't. The only difference is, during pregnancy, your desires may fluctuate much more dramatically. When you don't feel like having sex, you *really* don't even want to hear the word. Likewise, when desire strikes, you may feel you'd move a mountain to be with your partner. These wild fluctuations may be particularly prevalent in your first trimester, a time when hormones that are intimately linked to sexual desire can spin a bit out of control. In addition, don't be surprised if your newly developed maternal instincts also cause a bit of havoc with your sexual desires during the first trimester; experts say this too is a normal reaction.

"During pregnancy, not only is your body changing, but your newfound maternal feelings can trigger complex emotional responses," reports registered nurse and perinatal educator Joy Hacke. Suddenly, she says, motherhood and sexuality may seem "mutually exclusive," resulting in a temporary decrease in your sexual appetite during your first trimester. In at least one medical study of 112 pregnant Swedish couples in 1991, researchers found that a full 40 percent of women experienced at least some decline in their desire for sex for any number of assorted reasons during the first two to three months of their pregnancy.

Additionally, sometimes it may be you who is ready for sex, while your partner seems distant. This can be especially true if your pregnancy is a surprise. While it's a little like closing the barn door after the horse is already out, either partner may shy away from sex when a pregnancy is totally unexpected.

HOT AND HEAVY: YOUR SECOND TRIMESTER

Beginning somewhere around your fourteenth week of pregnancy, don't be surprised if you begin to feel a new surge of confidence and energy as well as a return of your sexual appetite. As many of the unpleasant symptoms of your first trimester (like morning sickness) begin to fade, you may find a whole new set of physiological changes occurring—at least some of which can have a positive effect on your desire for sex.

One of those changes involves an increase in blood volume, which in turn brings more circulation to your genitals. This can produce a swelling in your labia (the outside lips of your vulva) and in your clitoris, the area at the top of your vagina where sexual stimulation is most prominent. Thanks to soaring estrogen levels, which have now stabilized at a much higher than normal level, you may also have more vaginal lubrication. This, in turn, may leave you with a feeling of sexual "readiness" nearly all the time.

If your breasts are traditionally a focal point of sexual stimulation, you may experience some particularly pleasant changes and some welcome surprises during your second trimester. As your milk ducts develop, the tissue inside your breasts can become compressed, putting more pressure on sensitive nerve endings. This, in turn, can heighten your pleasure considerably whenever your breasts are touched or stroked. In addition, studies show that breast stimulation increases the production of the hormone oxytocin, the "biochemical of lust." And the higher your levels of oxytocin rise, the more desire you have for sex!

Don't be surprised, however, if you experience leaky breasts during sex—more specifically, a release of colostrum, the thin, yellow-tinged fluid that develops as a precursor to milk. While this might temporarily

Real Life

HOT SEX AND PRENATAL VITAMINS

Q: My sister is convinced that her prenatal vitamins increased her sexual appetite during pregnancy. I'm in my twelfth week and have no desire for sex. Her solution is to take more vitamins. Can this really help?

A: Your question is a good one—and it was exactly the same one on the minds of a group of Hungarian doctors in 1996. That's when they conducted a study of some 1,200 pregnant women to see if, in fact, prenatal vitamins could influence sexual activity during pregnancy. The research, published in the *British Journal of Obstetrics and Gynecology*, required half the pregnant women in the study to take a prenatal vitamin, while the other half took a placebo that contained only trace elements. The women then answered a roster of questions about their sexual activity, including how often they had intimate relations during each trimester. The end result: Both groups of women fared pretty much the same. The multivitamins, say the researchers, didn't appear to make any difference in their desire or enjoyment of sex.

That said, experts agree that because prenatal vitamins may help you avoid fatigue, you could simply feel more like having sex—which may have been the case with your sister. Also, ask when her sexual appetite kicked in. If it was during her second trimester, then chances are her hormones and other physiological events played a much larger role than the prenatal vitamins.

upset or even frighten you or your partner—or cause either one of you to momentarily feel turned off—remember that the leakage is normal, not dangerous to you, and not harmful to your partner, even if swallowed.

Finally, the position of your baby in your uterus during the second trimester can also create a pressure that actually enhances orgasm. This, combined with the increased blood flow to your genitals, might just allow you to climax in a way you never could before. If you had some difficulty achieving orgasm before pregnancy, you may even find that you are climaxing far more easily and more often during your second trimester.

If you had no problems climaxing before, you may find that you now are multiorgasmic. An encouraging survey result from some 17,000 women conducted by BabyCenter.com found that 36 percent of pregnant women reported better orgasms during pregnancy than ever before.

SEX AND YOUR THIRD TRIMESTER: WHAT YOU CAN EXPECT

While your second trimester may have been erotic bliss, don't be surprised if suddenly your desires decrease once again, usually beginning around your twenty-fourth or twenty-sixth week of pregnancy. Your growing tummy can present a real challenge to sexual comfort, while pain associated with increased weight—particularly backaches—can make it difficult to find a position where sex is comfortable, let alone erotic.

In addition, all that extra genital blood flow that made touch seem so pleasurable during your second trimester may now increase to such a degree that even being lightly stroked can be painful. The extra weight of your growing baby can leave you feeling fatigued too. Combined with a lack of sleep that can dominate the third trimester—not to mention feelings of unattractiveness that can prevail—sex may once again be the furthest thing from your mind. In that 1991 Swedish study mentioned earlier, researchers found that 75 percent of women had far less sexual desire during their third trimester.

Also remember, however, that when it comes to our sexual desires, *nothing* is ever cast in stone. A BabyCenter.com survey found that nearly 10 percent of some 17,000 women said they actually became a "sex machine" in their third trimester, and just couldn't get enough love! The point is that you shouldn't be surprised by any behavior or sexual feeling you develop during pregnancy—or by the fact that your desires may change from one week or even one day to the next. Any and all is considered normal.

Real Life

MORE ORGASMS, LESS SATISFACTION

Q: Throughout my entire pregnancy, sex has been just great—better than it was before pregnancy! But now that I'm in my third trimester, suddenly my orgasms don't feel the same—it's like I'm not really feeling satisfied, even with multiple orgasms or more sex. I'm afraid that maybe pregnancy has done something to my body, and I'll never be able to have a good orgasm again. Is this possible?

A: What you are experiencing is likely the result of conditions specifically related to the late stages of pregnancy and will probably cease soon after you give birth. For many women, orgasms that occur late in pregnancy don't appear to offer the same sense of relief as they did before— and as you pointed out, more sex isn't the answer, particularly since even multiple orgasms won't make much difference. Often the problem is related to the fact that there is so much pressure on your genitals near the end of pregnancy that in many ways your vagina is being continually stimulated, thereby reducing the effect of the orgasmic release. According to childbirth educator Robin Elise Weiss, while you may indeed not feel the same sense of relief from an orgasm during the final stage of your pregnancy, the experience can still be very pleasurable, particularly if you don't focus so intently on the end result. After your baby is born, your full feelings of satisfaction should return.

Sex, Your Partner, and Your Pregnancy

While the most dramatic pregnancy-related changes in sexual appetite clearly belong to women, it may surprise you to learn that men can also experience some degree of difference in their lusty appetite during each of your three trimesters.

Early on in your pregnancy, you may, for example, notice that your partner is far more interested in having sex than he ever was before. That's because, for many men, having bona fide proof that they can reproduce causes testosterone levels to soar, producing a masculinity boost—and an

Real Life

SEX, PAIN, AND PREGNANCY

Q: Is sex supposed to hurt during pregnancy—I mean, beyond a sense of general discomfort caused by my huge size? Whenever I have intercourse, I feel very irritated and very sore—and this has grown much worse now that I am in my third trimester. My doctor said it's nothing to worry about, but it is very uncomfortable and getting worse. Any suggestions?

A: Since you discussed this with your doctor, I am going to assume that you have been checked for any vaginal infections, such as yeast or bacterial vaginosis, both of which can cause the kind of irritation you describe. If you haven't been tested—and certainly if you have any other symptoms, including a cheesy white discharge or a yellow or gray or foul-smelling discharge, particularly after intercourse—talk to your doctor right away. That said, it's important to realize that as a pregnancy progresses, vaginal tissue frequently becomes irritated, particularly after long sessions of intimate contact. Although many women produce abundant lubrication during pregnancy, this is not always the case. In addition, if you are having a lot of sex, particularly long lovemaking sessions, the lubrication you do have may not be sufficient.

What can help is a non-inflammatory lubricant, such as Astroglide, SilkenSecret, or Slippery Stuff, all of which are approved for use during pregnancy. You should, however, abstain from sex until your vagina feels healed and no longer irritated. In addition, if you feel internal pressure during intercourse, experts say it is wise to avoid very deep penile penetration. You can also try changing the angle of your vagina by using pillows to elevate your hips and buttocks. Doing this will alter the way your partner enters your body, which may help reduce pressure and even some vaginal irritation.

increase in sex drive—second to none. Researcher and recognized parenting expert Armin Brott, author of *The Expectant Father*, reports that just having the knowledge that they *can* make a baby causes most men to feel an almost immediate desire to make *more* babies—a kind of evolutionary bias that ultimately translates into wanting sex a whole lot more, particularly in the days and weeks just following the confirmation of your conception.

In addition, many men report that they also feel much closer to their partners when they find out they are pregnant. Since for some men closeness can only be expressed erotically, it's not hard to see why sex can be foremost on their minds.

And while fears about sex and pregnancy hit men as well as women, for the most part, hesitations aren't likely to occur during the first trimester. That's because at this point in time, he can't see or feel any signs of your baby, so in many ways he's not connecting anything he does with you as affecting that child. That can change, however, when you enter your second trimester and your pregnancy starts to show. Don't be surprised if he suddenly turns from a raging tiger into a bit of a nurturing teddy bear, at least for a little while. Studies show that once a pregnancy becomes visible, some men develop a fear of having sex—afraid that their actions may somehow harm their partner or their baby. If you also feel some degree of fear, you may find that you feed off each other's anxieties, so much so that you end up avoiding sex through much of your pregnancy—even though it could be both pleasurable and healthy for you both.

There is also the possibility that your partner's disinterest in sex may be the result of other issues he has with you, or other problems in the relationship that have little or nothing to do with the fact that you are pregnant. This may be particularly true if your pregnancy came as a surprise and not something he was anticipating or looking forward to. While in many instances his negative feelings will pass on their own, sometimes it may require some serious discussions and/or the help of a counselor to sort things out. If this turns out to be the case for you, don't panic, and don't make the mistake of attributing everything to your pregnancy, failing to look at the deeper issues involved. The sooner you can tackle the problems, as they really are, the sooner they can be solved, and the better and happier your pregnancy will be. Conversely, letting things drag on while communication between the two of you drops off even more can only add to your anxiety and unhappiness.

SEX AND YOUR RELATIONSHIP: WHAT TO DO

Regardless of what is causing the problem, to help prevent sexual mis-communication from developing—or to stop it from growing worse—it's imperative that you and your partner continue to talk at all times. It's important that he knows how you feel, and it's important as well to encourage him to share his feelings with you, including his fears and desires. By communicating and sharing your feelings—not only about sex, but about parenting and especially about each other—neither of you will be as bothered or upset by whatever takes place during pregnancy.

Also important: Make certain your partner understands that the physical and emotional changes related to pregnancy are temporarily coloring some of your reactions as well. By keeping the lines of communication open, you can take the confusion out of your relationship and help ensure that your pregnancy remains happy and calm for both you and your partner.

Intimacy vs. Intercourse:
How to Stay Close Without Sex

For many couples, sex, particularly intercourse, will remain a vital and important part of the relationship throughout the pregnancy. For some women, however, sex may be so uncomfortable—or even medically ill advised—that intercourse is strictly off limits. While this can put a significant strain on your relationship, it doesn't have to. One way to ensure that it won't is to acknowledge that there are a wide array of activities that constitute "sex"—and they don't always have to include intercourse. Partner masturbation is one important way that you can both feel satisfied without intercourse. If orgasm is difficult for you—or if your doctor suggests you avoid it—then you can manually stimulate your partner, helping him to achieve climax, while you enjoy the physical closeness of intimate touching and caressing.

If, in fact, intercourse does become a problem for you at any time during your pregnancy, it's vital that you and your partner continue to have as much intimate contact as possible and that you not turn away from physical closeness. Hugging, kissing, holding hands, giving each

other back rubs and massages, even slow dancing in the dark to your favorite songs are all important ways to keep the intimacy alive throughout
your entire pregnancy, regardless of whether or not you participate in
more vigorous sexual activity.

And while this kind of intimate behavior is often second nature to
women, don't be surprised if it seems a bit difficult for your partner to
master, particularly at first. Remember, most men associate any physical
contact with the end goal of sexual intercourse. So, if you're pretty certain
that on any given day or night your actions and activities are not going
to wind up that way, you need to make your partner aware of that. Doing
so will help prevent any miscommunication that could leave him feeling
frustrated, hurt, or even rejected, and it will help take some of the pressure
off you to engage in something that, for whatever reason, doesn't feel right
to you at this time.

Finally, it's also important that you let your partner know that you
need to feel physically close and intimately connected throughout your
pregnancy, whether or not sex is involved. Make certain that he knows
how attractive he continues to be to you—extremely important if you are
not having much sex—and let him know how much it means that you
continue to have a close, intimate bond during your pregnancy. A few
well-chosen words in this direction can go a long way not only in helping your mate understand how you feel, but in heading off potential
problems while you encourage him to give you whatever level of care, attention, and intimate contact you want and need.

Sex and Pregnancy:
Overcoming the Six Most Common Fears

In the not-so-distant past, the words "sex" and "pregnancy" were barely
ever mentioned in the same sentence. Because pregnant women were often viewed as "fragile," rumors abounded on how sex would likely harm
them or the baby. And because the topic was so rarely discussed, not
much was done to squash these rumors. In fact, superstitions and half-
truths about the dangers of sex during pregnancy passed from one gener-
ation to the next for centuries.

Thankfully, however, change is taking place. Today even the conser-

Real Life

CONDOMS, SEX, AND PREGNANCY

Q: I read that if you use a condom while having sex during pregnancy, you can protect your baby, but my partner says this is not true, and he refuses to wear one. I'm scared to have sex without one—and he refuses to have sex with one—so nobody's having any fun. Is he right, or am I?

A: I don't know how much this is going to help you or your intimate life, but in some ways you are both right. First, and most important, if your partner has any risk of a sexually transmitted disease (STD)—if he has herpes, for example, or if he has sex outside of your relationship—then a condom is important and can help protect you from contracting any infection from him. While the mucous plug situated between your cervix and uterus blocks bacteria from reaching your baby during pregnancy, research shows that certain STDs—such as a herpes infection—can cause problems during delivery and affect your baby at that time. So, in this respect, if your partner's sexual activities *are at all in question,* then a condom is probably a very good idea. If, on the other hand, he's healthy and loyal, then his objections to condom use are justified.

There is, however, one more way a condom might help you enjoy sex more during pregnancy. For some pregnant women, sexual activity can bring on a harmless but painful bout of cramping, particularly if your partner ejaculates into your vagina. This is because certain chemicals found in semen can cause mild stimulation to the cervix, which in turn enhances the slight cramping that most women feel following sex during pregnancy. Using the condom will help keep this problem from happening. Your other option: that he simply withdraw his penis before ejaculation.

vative American College of Obstetricians and Gynecologists reports that as long as a woman is feeling good and the pregnancy is not in any jeopardy, she is free to have sex as much as she wants—right up until the day of delivery. Unfortunately, even with these encouraging words, old fears die hard—and many couples continue to experience unnecessary concern.

To help set the record straight and provide you with the very latest information available, what follows is a guide to **the six most common fears about sex during pregnancy.** With answers provided by some of the nation's top experts, the goal is to help you open a dialogue with your partner and with your doctor, so together you can determine what is a safe and appropriate level of sexual activity during *your* pregnancy.

FEAR #1: MISCARRIAGE

Although most doctors agree that sex won't cause a miscarriage in an otherwise healthy pregnancy, this fear remains high on the list of many couples. Most are especially fearful during the first trimester, when admittedly the threat of loss is always greatest. However, according to Dr. Diana Danilenko and colleagues at the Mayo Clinic, the most common causes of miscarriage are genetic factors and infections. If neither of these two conditions exists, she reports that sex isn't likely to cause you any problems. If these factors *are* present, you could miscarry anyway, whether you have sex or not. The bottom line: Don't be fearful, but always ask your doctor if your pregnancy is in any jeopardy and let her know you plan to continue your normal sex life.

FEAR #2: PREMATURE LABOR

Surveys show that among the most common fears couples experience in the second and especially the third trimester is premature labor. Throw sex into the mix, and those fears can soar. However, as early as 1993, at least one very large study involving more than 13,000 women found that preterm labor was *less common* among women who had intercourse at least once a week during their pregnancy. More recently, a 2001 study involving nearly 600 women and published in the journal *Obstetrics and Gynecology* found that sex during pregnancy was not only safe, it actually had a *protective* effect against early labor in all but a very small subgroup of women (those carrying more than one baby or suffering from placental problems). The researchers also reported a tiny increased risk among those couples who used the "male superior" position late in the third trimester—something that a few other studies have found as well.

The bottom line: If your pregnancy is healthy and you are not at risk for premature labor, then having sex clear through to the end is probably okay for you—particularly if you avoid the male-superior position (see "The Five Best Positions for Pregnant Sex" later in this chapter). If you do begin to experience extreme cramping after intercourse, talk to your doctor before you try again.

FEAR #3: HURTING THE BABY

In a study conducted at Memorial University of Newfoundland in 1999, more than half the mothers questioned believed that sex during pregnancy could harm their baby. Other research shows that many men share that fear. In reality, however, this should be the least of your pregnancy worries. According to Linda B. Jenkins, a registered nurse and childbirth educator from Lafayette, California, "It is virtually impossible to harm the fetus in the uterus." Experts from the Harvard Medical School concur, citing the fact that your baby literally floats in a pool of fluid inside your uterus—and that pool is protected by your abdominal wall and your entire pelvic structure. All of this serves to cushion your baby against everything but the most severe blows to your stomach. Dr. Danilenko also reminds us that because of both uterine muscle and amniotic fluid, your partner's penis has no chance of ever coming near the baby or causing any harm, even with deep penetration. In addition, your cervical mucous plug, which guards the opening of your uterus, prevents sperm and any bacteria from coming in contact with your baby, so there is no threat of danger here.

The bottom line: Sex won't harm your baby. And in case you're wondering if Junior will know what you and Dad are up to, the answer is no. While your baby will likely feel the sensations of your body moving, he or she won't know if you're dancing the tango, hanging curtains, or making love.

FEAR #4: BLEEDING AND CRAMPING

One of the most disconcerting events is to develop cramping, or especially bleeding, during pregnancy, particularly when it follows sex. In truth, however, with or without sex, bleeding in early pregnancy occurs in as many as half of all women, and for over 60 percent there are no serious problems. Among the most common reasons is a fragile cervix.

"Because the entire genital region begins to become blood filled, the cervix also becomes more vascular," says childbirth educator Robin Elise Weiss. Because the cervix descends lower into the vagina during pregnancy, the tiny capillaries lining the surface can sometimes break during intercourse. The result can be a very small amount of spotting somewhere between ten and sixty minutes following intercourse.

In addition, with or without orgasm (see more about this below), many women also experience mild uterine contractions following sexual stimulation. Similar to Braxton-Hicks contractions, which occur spontaneously throughout pregnancy, cramping following sex is not the same as labor contractions. "Generally these contractions rarely last more than an hour after [sex] and are generally not considered dangerous," says Weiss.

The bottom line: If mild cramping or bleeding does develop following sex, experts from Harvard Medical School advise resting an hour or two in bed, during which time symptoms should subside. If they don't, or if cramping or bleeding is severe, call your doctor before having any further sexual activity. (See the red flags for pregnant sex below.) And always mention any bleeding to your doctor, no matter how slight.

FEAR #5: ORGASM

Because orgasm can generally result in some level of cramping and even a small amount of spotting, many women are frightened about climaxing during pregnancy. For the most part, however, these fears are unfounded. In the same study on premature labor reported in *Obstetrics and Gynecology* in 2001, researchers found that orgasm occurring late in pregnancy, with or without intercourse, appeared to *reduce* the risk of preterm delivery. Two previous studies, conducted in 1980 and 1984, found a similar result. The bottom line: While orgasms do cause your uterus to contract, those contractions do not result in cervical dilation, and that's why they won't initiate labor. And while your baby has no idea what is going on during sexual activity, doctors say they do experience a euphoric-like hormonal rush when you have an orgasm. Again, do mention any bleeding or cramping to your doctor.

FEAR #6: ORAL/ANAL SEX

While in theory, oral or anal sex might seem safer than intercourse, many couples aren't certain, and some are even frightened that it could cause even greater problems. In reality, the only real dangers associated with oral sex is if your partner has cold sores on or around the lips, or if he harbors any oral or dental infections, including thrush. If so, these infections can be transmitted to you and may interfere with your pregnancy and/or your delivery. Likewise, you should not perform oral sex on a partner who has any evidence of a sexually transmitted disease or does not know if he has been exposed to an STD. One last caution: There should be no blowing into your vagina during oral sex. Doing so can cause an air embolism, or air bubble, sometimes powerful enough to block a blood vessel, resulting in death for you and your baby.

When it comes to anal sex, most doctors agree that if this is something you have done before, continuing during pregnancy is not going to cause any harm to your baby. It could, however, be painful for you if you suffer with hemorrhoids. If you have not tried anal sex in the past, it's probably not a good idea to try it for the first time during pregnancy. There can be some minor tissue tearing associated with this practice, which may be more intense if it occurs for the first time during pregnancy. Still, this probably would pose no harm to the baby. The bottom line: Neither sexual practice is likely to interfere with your pregnancy, but get your doctor's okay before you try.

Safe and Healthy Pregnant Sex: What to Do Right Now

As safe and as healthy as sex can be during pregnancy, there are times and situations when it's not going to be a good idea. For some women, prob-

Real Life

SEX AND LABOR INDUCTION

Q: When my best friend went past her due date, her doctor told her to have sex to bring on labor. She did, labor started, and she delivered about ten hours afterward. Can sex really bring on labor? And if so, then why is it considered safe to have sex during pregnancy?

A: First, it's important to separate the effects of sex during the course of pregnancy from sex at the very end of pregnancy, when it's time for baby to be born. If your cervix is *not dilated*, as it is not likely to be during pregnancy, then no matter what the activity, it won't encourage labor. If, on the other hand, your cervix has begun to dilate—meaning baby is ready to be born—any physical activity, whether walking or having sex, can help kick off the uterine contractions that officially launch labor. In addition, however, when you have an orgasm, you release oxytocin—a powerful chemical that not only accounts for pleasurable feelings, but also stimulates uterine contractions. Your partner's semen contains chemicals called prostaglandins, which, when released in your vagina *after cervical dilation* has started, can also encourage contractions. That said, a recent meta-analysis of all available medical literature on the subject has led doctors from the Royal College of Obstetrics in London to conclude that there is no clear-cut medical evidence that sex affects labor one way or the other. Still, because it can't hurt, many doctors continue to recommend it. If nothing else, it can help you to relax and take your mind off the fact that you are overdue!

lems can develop right at the start of pregnancy, making even first-trimester sex a risky venture. For others, the second or third trimester may bring the greatest risks.

In any event, if your doctor determines that sex might be a problem, you should heed his or her advice and abstain. However, you should also make certain that you clearly understand your doctor's instructions, including why sexual activity is being limited and *for how long*. Often a doctor may tell a woman to refrain from sex, particularly if she's reported an episode of bleeding or cramping. While the woman may take this to mean "refrain from sex throughout your pregnancy," the doctor may have meant only to take a rest for a week or ten days.

That said, make sure you always get your doctor's advice on sex if any of the following red flags exist:

✓ Vaginal bleeding, in any amount, at any time during your pregnancy. While light spotting is often a normal part of pregnancy, particularly following intercourse, leave it to your doctor to decide what it means for you.

✓ If you are diagnosed with an incompetent cervix. In this condition your cervix dilates prematurely, which can increase the risk of premature labor or even miscarriage.

✓ If you are at any increased risk for preterm labor, particularly if you delivered prematurely in a previous pregnancy.

✓ If you are diagnosed with placenta previa, a condition in which the placental sac, which holds and supports your baby during pregnancy, slips downward to cover a portion of your cervical opening. This, in turn, may increase the risk of early cervical dilation and premature labor, both of which can sometimes be aggravated by sexual stimulation.

✓ Anytime you are carrying more than one baby. In this case, you may have to refrain from intercourse starting late in your second trimester and into the start of your third trimester. In some instances, your doctor may extend or renew the "no intercourse" orders in the final weeks of your pregnancy to help ensure against early labor and give your babies as much developmental time in your uterus as is possible.

Real Life

MASTURBATION, VIBRATORS, AND PREGNANCY

Q: My husband is working two jobs to help us afford this baby, but the problem is I don't see him very often. Sometimes I'm really in the mood for sex, and he's not here. I'm wondering if masturbation is safe during pregnancy and if I could use my vibrator to achieve orgasm.

A: Generally, anything you can safely do with a partner, you can safely do on your own—so yes, masturbation is considered a very safe way to achieve sexual satisfaction during pregnancy. In fact, if, for any reason, intercourse is difficult for you during this time, experts say partner masturbation can be a wonderful release for the both of you. As to the vibrator, there are no studies to show it can be a problem—so long as it's kept very clean. However, if it is a very powerful vibrator—giving you more uterine activity than intercourse would—then it's a good idea to check with your doctor first. This is a general rule of thumb whenever you place anything in your vagina during pregnancy, including sex toys or even lubricants.

The Five Best Positions for Pregnant Sex

While sex may be considered safe and even pleasurable during pregnancy, clearly, it's not always going to be comfortable. Your increasing size, along with other comfort issues, can make intercourse difficult, painful, or even seem impossible, particularly in the later stages of your pregnancy.

What can help is choosing positions that do not cause you to lie flat on your back or have your partner's weight directly on your abdomen. This is particularly important advice in your second and third trimesters, since doctors advise that you should not lie on your back after the twentieth week of pregnancy.

So, if you've ever thought about experimenting with some new and different sexual positions, pregnancy may be the right time to start! While you don't want to try anything that would put your body in dangerous or painful positions, you can feel free to use your imagination to find the variations that suit you and your partner best. To help you get started, a number of sex education experts, including Dr. Pepper Schwartz and the grande dame of sexual education, Dr. Ruth Westheimer, report that the following positions could make pregnant sex easier and more pleasurable for you and your partner.

1. SPOONING

In this position, you lie on your left side, your body curled in a C position, with knees drawn up and arms in front. Your partner, who should be facing your back, mimics the position, curling or "spooning" around you. His arms can go around your body, so he is free to touch your breasts or your vagina. For intercourse he enters your vagina from behind, while both of you remain lying on your left side.

2. SIDE BY SIDE

In this variation, you lie on your left side facing your partner, who is lying on his right side. He slips one leg over yours (your leg can be straight or bent), which allows him to enter your vagina at an angle. Not only will this help keep his weight off your tummy, it also enables him to control the thrust of his entry, which in turn may be more comfortable for you. This position can be very helpful if you are experiencing any vaginal irritation during intercourse or if you have any mild to moderate pain during sex.

3. WOMAN ON TOP

Here entry is through the front of your vagina; the only thing different is that your partner lies flat on his back, while you perch over him. Since lying facedown may be difficult, many women find it much more comfortable simply to straddle their partner and remain in a semi-sitting position. This posture also enables you to control the thrust of your partner's penis, which may help make intercourse more comfortable for you.

4. EDGE OF THE BED

This position can be very comfortable in the late stages of pregnancy, when even lying on your side becomes difficult. Here you begin by sitting on the edge of the bed, legs spread, with both feet planted on the floor. Then you slowly lower the upper half of your body back onto the bed, keeping your buttocks as close to the edge of the mattress as possible. For intercourse, your partner can stand or bend over you, with entry through the front of your vagina. Because this position allows your partner the deepest and most penetrating thrust power, be careful you don't experience any pain. If thrusting does become too hard—and listen to your body on this one—then your partner can simply pull back so he does not penetrate you as deeply.

5. HANDS AND KNEES

In this position, you begin by kneeling, the calves of your legs tucked under your thighs. Then rise up slightly—enough to stretch your arms out and put the palms of your hands down on the bed. Your final position will have your face, your breasts, and the front of your tummy facing the bed, while your knees and the palms of your hands touch the bed. Your partner enters your vagina from behind. To help stimulate you, his hands can wrap around your body, cupping your breasts and stimulating your genitals. This is the best position to allow for manual stimulation and may increase your chance of a multiple orgasm.

Sex, Love, and the Safety of Your Pregnancy: A Final Word

While sex may not be the first thing on your mind during pregnancy, try to remember that a warm, nurturing, intimate relationship can not only put that wonderful "glow" in your cheeks, it may also help draw you and your partner closer together. Staying physically close during pregnancy can also go a long way in establishing the fact that becoming parents doesn't have to mean you must stop being lovers—a concept that can help you to resume your sexual relationship more easily after baby is born. Later, in Chapter 12, you will also find some new information on sex after childbirth—including what you can expect from yourself and your partner.

Right now, however, the main thing is to keep the lines of communication open and the commitment to each other strong, whether sex is involved or not. Doing so can help you have a happier, healthier pregnancy and may even influence how quickly and easily you bounce back after giving birth.

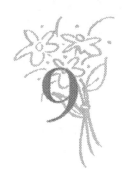

Your Pregnancy
from Nine to Five

*What Every Working
Mother-to-Be Must Know*

Once upon a time, the idea of a woman working through her pregnancy was practically unheard of. Not so anymore. Today more than 1 million women in the U.S. workforce get pregnant each year, and up to 90 percent work well into their third trimester.

While for some, the transition from working woman to working mother-to-be is a smooth and easy one, for many there can be more than a few bumps in the road. As you strive to integrate your professional persona into the ever-increasing physical and psychological demands of pregnancy, your working life may become a bit more complex than you thought it would. While female coworkers may be clamoring for the most intimate details of your pregnancy, the men in your work environment may have the exact opposite reaction. Often they may be too embarrassed even to acknowledge your pregnancy, and some may even pull back from you professionally, fearful of asking you to participate in things that normally would be a routine part of your job.

While you may be eager to share some of your excitement about your pregnancy with some coworkers or even your boss, don't be surprised if their attitude leaves you feeling that you have to constantly monitor that enthusiasm. Many professional women report feeling fearful that expressing too much excitement about their baby will be interpreted as being less interested in their work—and ultimately being less interested in coming *back* to work after their baby is born.

To compensate, you may even find yourself going way overboard in the opposite direction—downplaying your pregnancy or even trying to ignore it, while working longer hours and getting projects in sooner than you normally would. The temptation is definitely there to beat your own record for speed and endurance, simply trying to prove that your job is as important to you as your baby.

If this is starting to sound familiar, it's important that you stop, take a breath, and recognize and acknowledge your feelings. And, from time to time, take a step back to look at what's really going on in your professional life. Ask yourself if it's really necessary to do all you are doing—or are you just trying to show the world that pregnancy won't stop you?

Also important is to recognize that, like it or not, being pregnant *is* going to put some limitations on what you may be able to accomplish professionally until your baby is born. Certainly first-trimester problems, such as morning sickness or fatigue, can mean that you'll miss a meeting or two or that you simply *can't* take work home over the weekend as you normally might. Depending on the type of job you have, as your pregnancy progresses, the physical demands of your growing baby can make it more difficult to perform certain work tasks or do them as quickly or efficiently as you might.

The point is, you must acknowledge your pregnancy and accept that there will be some limitations beyond your control. And that your professional life won't come to a screeching halt because of it. While pushing yourself to extremes trying to compensate may be tempting, doing so is not only going to complicate your pregnancy, it is also likely to take you further away from achieving your professional goals. If ever there was a time to reflect on all you have accomplished in your professional life and recognize that you are more than the sum of today's assignments, it is now!

In addition, you can also ease some of your boss's fears by assuring him or her that your plan is to work through as much of your pregnancy as possible and to return to your job after baby is born. By taking the time to reiterate your commitment not only to the company, but to your own career goals, you'll ease everyone's mind and further cement your place at work.

Working Decisions: What You Must Consider

Whether you *want* to continue working for personal or professional reasons or finances dictate that you *must*, it's important to recognize that at times certain pregnancy-related health considerations might preclude your wants or your needs. There are a number of factors you must consider before deciding whether to work through all or even part of your pregnancy. And this is one decision you definitely should not make alone. According to experts from the American College of Obstetricians and Gynecologists, it's imperative that you discuss your job intentions with your physician before deciding what to do.

When having that talk, make certain that your doctor understands your job requirements, including not only the physical tasks involved in your work (such as standing for long periods of time, working at a desk, lifting heavy objects, etc.), but also the level of emotional stress you generally experience on the job. Why is this so important? Studies published in the May 2002 journal of *Epidemiology* revealed that women exposed to both physical and mental stress while working can increase their risk of preeclampsia—a dangerous form of pregnancy-related high blood pressure—by up to five times that of women who stay at home during pregnancy.

In addition, be sure to tell your doctor about your commute to work. Do you drive, or take a bus or a train, and is your commute longer than thirty minutes? Do you frequently have to stand on crowded public transportation? Your doctor will use your answers to these questions, as well as the specific factors about your job, to assess any work-related pregnancy risks and advise you on how to proceed.

Work and Your Health

Besides your job tasks, how you actually feel while you are pregnant will play a big role in deciding whether you can—or should—continue working. Do you have the energy to do your job? Are you sidelined by extreme morning sickness, nausea, or vomiting? Are you plagued with bleeding problems, cramping, high blood pressure, or high blood sugar? Any or all of these factors must be taken into consideration when deciding whether to work through your pregnancy.

Other important factors you and your doctor should consider:

✓ Previous health and pregnancy history

✓ Any evidence of a weak cervix

✓ Previous premature labor problems

✓ Any severe back, leg, or circulation problems

✓ Past history of premature rupture of membranes

✓ Personal history of heart or kidney disease

In most instances, your doctor will work with you to help ensure that you can safely continue your job duties through part or all of your pregnancy. However, if your physician suggests that you stop working, do heed the advice—but make certain you understand the reason behind the recommendation. Doing so will help ensure that you don't endanger your pregnancy while at home.

Workplace Hazards: What You Need to Know

In addition to your personal health factors, there are also some job-related hazards you must consider. For most women, these include dangers related to specific job tasks, such as heavy lifting, bending, standing or sitting for long periods of time, as well as dangers related to the work environment. This would include any exposure to questionable chemicals, poor air circulation, or ergonomic issues, such as the kind of chair you are required to use or the motions involved in a specific work task.

The good news here is that very few jobs pose hazards serious enough to threaten the health of you or your baby, and those that do often can be altered to accommodate your needs. Perhaps most important is the fact that there are laws in place to *ensure* your right to work in a safe environment during pregnancy—legislation you'll learn more about later in this chapter.

In the meantime, experts from the American College of Obstetricians and Gynecologists and the March of Dimes offer the following points to consider when making safety assessments of your workplace, along with some *pregnancy-friendly* changes that can help.

FACTOR # 1: EXPOSURE TO HAZARDOUS SUBSTANCES

This area of concern includes any job tasks that cause you to come into contact with metals or chemicals that could be harmful to you or your baby. The most prominent on the list include mercury and lead, which can be part of other products, such as solvents. Depending on your level of exposure and the length of time you are exposed, problems can include preterm delivery and smaller babies.

For a More Pregnancy-Friendly Workplace: If your job requires direct contact with any potentially dangerous substance or if any chemical causes you to feel ill during pregnancy, ask to be reassigned to a job task where there is less or no exposure to the offending substances. Even if these substances merely are present in your direct environment, and you don't handle them directly, you should ask to be reassigned to an area where exposure is minimized. Remember: You cannot be turned down or penalized for requesting changes based on threats to your health or your baby's health. (See "Pregnancy and the Law" later in this chapter.)

FACTOR #2: ENVIRONMENTAL NOISE

The level of noise you are exposed to during your pregnancy can be linked to hearing loss in your baby, and it can also increase the risk of low birthweight and preterm delivery. In one study, children with high-frequency hearing loss were more commonly born to mothers who experienced noise between 85 and 95 decibels daily during pregnancy. According to the U.S. Environmental Protection Agency, regular exposure to 44 to 55 decibels of sound is considered very safe for the general public, while neonatal intensive care units restrict their noise levels to 45 decibels or below. Normal conversation clocks in between 55 and 60 decibels (depending on who's doing the talking!), while a whisper is about 30 decibels. By comparison, power mowers generate anywhere from 65 to 95 decibels depending on the size. As such, if you work in close proximity to any machinery that continually runs at 55 decibels or higher, you could be putting your baby at risk.

For a More Pregnancy-Friendly Workplace: Most important is that you request to be moved to an area where noise is minimal. To further reduce risks, talk to your employer about purchasing hearing protection devices. Resembling headphones, they are designed to dramatically reduce assaults on your ears. Since noise is absorbed through the womb, this obviously won't affect what does get through to your baby. However, it can help cut down on some of the physiological reactions to noise that occur in your body, which may provide a small help to your baby and a major help to you.

FACTOR #3: EXPOSURE TO VIRUSES AND INFECTIONS

If you work in the healthcare profession, as a schoolteacher, in a day care center, or even in a close office environment, catching any kind of "bug" is more likely; even colds spread more easily in close quarters. The viruses and infections you need to be especially mindful of include chicken pox, cytomegalovirus, hepatitis, herpes, rubella, and toxoplasmosis, all of which can significantly threaten the health of your pregnancy.

For a More Pregnancy-Friendly Workplace: Whenever possible, limit contact with any individual suspected of having any of these infections, including children; wash your hands frequently, particularly before and after using the rest room and before eating; talk to your doctor about whether certain vaccinations may help protect you. See Chapter 11 for more information and more precautions.

FACTOR #4: EXPOSURE TO RADIATION OR ANESTHESIA

Primarily a concern for those in the healthcare professions, exposure to either of these factors on a daily or regular basis can increase your risk of miscarriage, birth defects, or even cancer. You should also avoid contact with certain treatments, particularly the chemotherapy agents methotrexate and aminopterin, which have been linked to pregnancy risks.

For a More Pregnancy-Friendly Workplace: Ask for reassignment to an area of the hospital or clinic where you have no direct contact with these substances. If that is not possible, request that particular duties involving the administration of, or contact with, these substances be reassigned to someone else, and offer to swap duties with a coworker to minimize your risks.

FACTOR #5: VENTILATION OF WORK SPACE

Proper ventilation can be particularly important if your work involves the use of chemicals, solvents, or substances like foam, which cause an off-gassing—the release of potentially toxic chemicals into the immediate environment. Proper ventilation is also necessary if your work space contains pressed-wood furniture, carpeting, or drapes, which can also off-gas noxious chemicals such as formaldehyde.

According to doctors from the University of Michigan Health Center, the temperature of your work environment could be a problem too, particularly heat. Indeed, many pregnant women suffer dizzy spells or even fainting episodes when an environment is too warm—problems that can increase work-related injuries.

Real Life

COMPUTERS, CELLS PHONES, AND PREGNANCY RISKS

Q: My wife works at home in front of a computer all day long, plus she's constantly on her cell phone. I'm concerned that she may be exposing herself to too much radiation and hurting herself or our baby in the process. But she's convinced there's nothing wrong with using this equipment. Who's right?

A: It looks as if mother knows best—at least based on what we know so far. There is, in fact, no solid medical research to show that working in front of a computer or using a cell phone has any negative effects on pregnancy. Yet it's only fair to say that many doctors believe the safety data we do have is insufficient and that there *may* be problems associated with use. While computers don't give off any dangerous radiation, they do create an electromagnetic field around them—which some doctors say eventually may be recognized as having some effect on preg-

For a More Pregnancy-Friendly Workplace: Ask for relocation to the area of the building where ventilation is best. You can also request that a portable circulation fan or air cleaner be placed in your immediate environment, and you can seek reimbursement for a personal air cleaner to be kept on or near your desk. In addition, make your heat sensitivity known and tell your supervisor if your work area is too hot, whether it is winter or summer.

The Three Most Common Job Risks and How to Fix Them

In addition to whatever environmental factors may be compromising your pregnancy health, certain occupations can increase your risk of problems no matter where the activities are carried out.

The positions you assume while working—standing, sitting, or

nancy. Currently, there are reports of miscarriage clusters among women who work on computers or in an environment where lots of computers are used. To play it safe, many medical experts now recommend that a pregnant woman sit at arm's length from her computer monitor and at least three feet from the back of any other monitor used in her presence. If you are still concerned, or if sitting that far from the screen is not practical, then you can invest in a protective anti-radiation, anti-glare screen to attach to the front of the monitor. Another option is to purchase an ultra-thin flat panel monitor, or a notebook computer, which is generally not associated with as many risks.

In terms of cell phones, there is no firm evidence linking their use to any birth defects or other pregnancy problems in humans. However, a recent French study detailed how 6,000 baby chicks exposed to radiation emissions from cell phones were five times less likely to survive than a control group. Again, to err on the side of caution, using a wireless speakerphone or a headphone attached by wire to the cell phone can virtually eliminate all threat of problems. (See Chapter 10 for more information.)

bending, for example—can lead to significant discomfort. Sometimes the movements involved in the job task itself—including keystrokes associated with computer work—can cause problems during pregnancy as well. The good news is that, in most instances, there are simple modifications that you can make to help increase the safety of almost any job activity and make the tasks safer and more comfortable to perform during pregnancy.

According to registered nurse Judith Webster and Dr. R. Michael Morse of the Workcare Group, here's what to look out for and what you might try to change.

RISK #1: STANDING FOR LONG PERIODS OF TIME

If your job involves sales, cooking, nursing, waitressing, bartending, or any activity that keeps you on your feet most or all of your workday, you could be compromising your circulation and reducing your baby's supply of nutrients.

For a Safer Pregnancy: Reduce time on your feet by swapping job tasks with a coworker, even for just a few hours. The next best thing is to take a sitting break every twenty minutes, elevating your feet for five minutes while you rest. You can also try walking in place to exercise calf muscles and promote better circulation. If you must stand in one position, try placing one foot on a low step stool, which can help relieve back pressure and also help circulation.

RISK #2: LIFTING, BENDING, CLIMBING

Heavy lifting is most dangerous in your first trimester, when the risk of miscarriage is greatest, and in your third trimester, when the risk of premature labor is greatest. Since balance is sometimes compromised during your third trimester, any tasks involving climbing or using a ladder late in your pregnancy could increase your risk of a dangerous fall.

For a Safer Pregnancy: Avoid job tasks that involve lifting; if you can't, then reduce the load of what you lift by 25 percent or more each trimester. Ask about splitting or alternating risky tasks with another worker whose job doesn't entail such extreme motions.

RISK #3: SITTING FOR LONG PERIODS

Like standing in one spot too long, sitting in one position for an extended period can cause circulation problems as well as increase your risk of backaches.

For a Safer Pregnancy: Take hourly breaks that allow you to walk around for at least two minutes. Whenever possible, elevate your feet while sitting, using a small step stool or stack of telephone books under your desk. Several times an hour extend your legs, point your toes, and flex your feet. If your back is feeling stiff or sore, use a pillow to support the lower portion or invest in an ergonomic curved back pillow or one that contains a

> ## Real Life
>
> ### PLANES, TRAINS, BUSES, AND PREGNANCY HEALTH
>
> **Q:** I do a significant amount of long-distance traveling in my job—sometimes by plane, sometimes by train. In fact, I'm on the road at least two weeks out of every month. I'm wondering if this is going to be safe now that I'm pregnant, and if there are any health risks I should know about, particularly as my pregnancy progresses.
>
> **A:** Most experts agree that travel, in and of itself, is not harmful during pregnancy, particularly by train or bus. While air travel was once considered a little risky—mostly because of radiation caused by high-altitude flying—even that has been given a clean bill of health. Late in 2001, the American College of Obstetricians and Gynecologists issued a special advisory on air travel and pregnancy. They gave their stamp of approval for pregnant women to fly domestically until their thirty-sixth week of pregnancy, and internationally until the thirty-fifth week, providing the mother is in good health with no pregnancy complications. They do, however, advise extreme caution concerning air travel if a woman suffers with pregnancy-induced high blood pressure, poorly controlled gestational diabetes, sickle cell disease, or any health problem that might result in what is termed an "unforseen emergency." The advisory cautions against air travel for any woman at significant risk for premature labor or placental abnormalities. For more information on flying during pregnancy, see Chapter 10.

battery-operated massage mechanism. Also important: Avoid crossing your legs while sitting, which can decrease circulation.

Pregnancy and the Law: What You Need to Know

While you and your doctor may have decided it's safe for you to work, it's also going to take the cooperation of your employer if you are to continue your job during pregnancy. Fortunately, since the late 1970s, some im-

portant legislation has been put in place to ensure the ultimate cooperation from your place of business. Many company handbooks now clearly
spell out both the employers' obligations to women and women's rights
during pregnancy, all according to law.

Other employers, however, may not be so forthcoming about what
they are required to do for you, particularly when it comes to maternity
leave or insurance coverage. Some bosses may even try to dissuade you
from working during pregnancy or threaten you with job loss if you don't
do things exactly as they say. Therefore, it is imperative that you familiarize yourself with some of the basic legislation that is in place to protect
your rights as a pregnant working woman. To help you get started, here's
a quick primer on the four most important rulings you need to know.

PROTECTION #1: THE PREGNANCY DISCRIMINATION ACT

Passed in 1978, this legislation offers certain protections if you are unable
to work during part or all of your pregnancy, including the period just after you give birth. The main gist of this law is that it establishes certain
pregnancy problems as a disability—meaning that, as a worker, you are
entitled to the same coverage provided to any other employee, male or female, who suffers a disability that keeps him or her from working.

If your company employs fifteen people or more, your specific rights
include:

- Disability pay equal to that of a worker who takes a medical
  leave for any reason, such as a heart attack or a broken leg. If
  other workers are offered the chance to do a lighter or more
  suitable job during the time they are disabled, you are
  guaranteed this same right.

- The right to have your job held open the same amount of time
  your employer would hold a position for any employee suffering
  a disability.

- Your right to the same level of health insurance as all other
  employees, without changes to your deductible.

This legislation also protects against various forms of workplace discrimination based on your pregnancy status. For example:

- You cannot be refused a job or fired from a job simply because you are pregnant.

- You cannot be forced to stop working while pregnant—as long as you can physically perform your job tasks.

- Your employer cannot dictate the amount of time you must take off, either before or after your delivery.

- Regardless of any pregnancy-related time off, you are entitled to retain all seniority, retirement, and any other time-accrued benefits.

PROTECTION #2: THE FAMILY AND MEDICAL LEAVE ACT

Effective since 1993, and administered and enforced by the U.S. Department of Labor, this legislation entitles either men or women working for a company that employs fifty people or more to take up to twelve weeks of unpaid leave each year to deal with family health problems or crises. In terms of your pregnancy, this law affects your maternity leave by splitting it into two separate parts.

The first part, technically called a "medical leave," kicks in should your pregnancy or your postpartum recovery period physically keep you from doing your job. Your medical leave should be covered by the same disability insurance payments that are offered to others in your company who cannot work due to health problems. This part of the legislation also ensures your right to take time off to tend to any medical concern that may arise during your pregnancy, such as the need for an amniocentesis or ultrasound exam. Again, your time off should be covered by disability insurance payments, even if you miss only one or two days of work.

The second part of this law covers what is technically called "family leave" and deals with your right to stay home and care for your new baby even if you are physically able to work. Your total amount of leave time

An Expert's Opinion on

PREGNANCY DISABILITY

For the most part, your pregnancy will be healthy, and it's not likely you will need the disability protection provided by the Pregnancy Discrimination Act. However, if you do, it's important to understand what constitutes a pregnancy disability and what entitles you to protection under this legislation.

According to the experts at the American College of Obstetricians and Gynecologists, pregnancy disabilities fall into one of the following three categories:

1. *Disability caused by the pregnancy itself.* This includes problems such as nausea, vomiting, extreme fatigue, dizziness, or swollen legs and ankles. Because these symptoms are often short-lived or occur for only a short period of time, they are often considered a short-term disability. Giving birth is also considered a short-term disability, a fact that can influence how your company orchestrates your maternity leave—something you'll learn more about in a few minutes.

is twelve weeks, and you are free to split that in any way you like—taking off the first six weeks after giving birth, for example, then returning to work for two or three months, and taking an additional six weeks later in the year. Be aware, however, that your employer may require that you use your paid leave time first, including sick days, personal days, vacation time, disability leave time, or other accumulated time off, to take care of family concerns before asking for your official unpaid family leave time.

However you choose to distribute your leave time, it's important to know that your employer must continue to pay your health insurance. And unless you are considered a key company executive, your job position must be held open, providing you return on or before the conclusion of your twelve-week leave. One caveat: If you and your spouse work for the same company, you are only entitled to a *combined* twelve weeks of

2. *Disability linked to pregnancy complications.* This category includes rare but severe problems such as infection, bleeding, premature labor, or premature rupture of your amniotic sac. Also included are health problems you had prior to getting pregnant that might have disabling effects now, such as heart disease, diabetes, or high blood pressure.

3. *Disability due to job exposures.* This category covers any factors related to your job that can potentially harm your baby, such as an environment that is laden with potentially harmful chemicals, extremely loud noise, very hot or very cold temperatures, or odors that cause you to feel sick.

If your doctor decides that your pregnancy is disabling you in any way, he or she must put that in writing, and you should submit the letter to your employer. If your employer suggests that you stop working, but your doctor says it's okay to continue, it's smart to get that in writing from your physician.

family leave time. And remember, your company must regularly employ fifty people or more to be covered by this act.

For more specific information on the Family Leave Act, call the offices of the U.S. Equal Employment Opportunity Commission toll free at 800-669-4000, or visit them on the Internet at www.eeoc.gov.

PROTECTION #3: HEALTH INSURANCE PORTABILITY AND ACCOUNTABILITY ACT

Signed into action by President Bill Clinton in 1996, this legislation offers protection if you or your spouse should switch jobs and consequently health insurance plans while you are pregnant or if you enroll in a plan after conceiving. It guarantees that your healthcare needs, and the needs of your baby after birth, will be covered under any health insurance benefits plan, even if you or your employer should switch plans in the middle

HOW TO GIVE NOTICE FOR FAMILY LEAVE

Unless your time off is the result of an emergency situation, you are obligated to give your employer thirty days' notice of your intention to invoke the Family Leave Act. The Department of Labor provides Form WH-380 for this purpose. You can obtain a copy by calling your local Department of Labor office, or you can download it directly from the Internet at www.dol.gov/libraryforms/index.asp. If you do not give your employer the appropriate notice, the company does not have to grant you family leave, so it is in your best interest to obtain the form, fill it out completely, and submit it on time.

or even near the end of your pregnancy. If you should have to apply for coverage with a new insurer, you cannot be turned down based on the fact that you are pregnant.

Also important to note:

- Should your existing insurance be canceled or dropped due to an employment change, you have just sixty-three days in which to apply for any new insurance and still maintain protection under this law.

- If you were covered under your spouse's insurance and he loses that coverage for any reason, your employer must give you the right to join any group health insurance plan in effect in your place of business, as long as you do so within thirty days of losing your previous coverage.

- Your newborn cannot be denied medical coverage, regardless of when you joined your insurance plan, as long as you sign him or her up within thirty days of birth.

For more information on the protection offered you by this legislation, visit the Health Care Financing Administration on the Internet at www.hcfa.gov/medicaid/hipaa/online/000021.asp. Or you can call your local state Labor Department.

PROTECTION #4: OCCUPATIONAL SAFETY AND HEALTH ACT

This legislation requires your employer to provide a workplace that is free of any known hazards likely to cause serious harm to you or your baby. The act pertains not only to your specific job duties, but also to any chemicals or tools involved in your work. Should your job put your health in any danger, your employer is required by law to make you aware of those risks in writing. You may be surprised to learn that this legislation also includes dangers caused by ergonomic hazards—for example, chairs, desks, and computer equipment—that cause your body undue stress when used during pregnancy. The Occupational Safety and Health Administration (OSHA), which administers this act, could become your strongest ally should any health-related problems occur in conjunction with your work environment. OSHA is also available to do on-site inspections of work conditions at an *employee's request* to help guarantee safety standards, so don't be afraid to ask for help if you believe your job may be putting you or your baby at risk. Remember, legally, you cannot be penalized by your employer for asserting your rights—even if no violations are found. If, in fact, OSHA does discover that health or safety problems exist, your employer is bound by law to correct the situation and to keep you from further exposure to anything that is known to be potentially harmful to you or your baby. To contact OSHA, look up your local state office in the government listings of your phone book, or visit the website at www.osha.gov.

A second organization that can provide help in this area is the National Institute for Occupational Safety and Health (NIOSH), a division of the Centers for Disease Control. It can be very helpful in tracking down and correcting any health threats that may exist at your workplace while you are pregnant or at any time. To contact NIOSH, call 800-35-NIOSH, or visit the website at www.cdc.gov/niosh.

Real Life

BREAST-FEEDING ON THE JOB

Q: I plan to nurse my baby after she is born, but I just found out that my workplace does not offer any private areas (other than the ladies' room) or any break time for me to express milk or to nurse my baby even if my nanny brings her to the premises. Are there any laws that can help me fight what seems like discrimination?

A: Unless you live in Connecticut, Hawaii, Minnesota, or Illinois—the only states where legislation requires employers to allot certain rights to breast-feeding mothers—you are limited to the generosity of your employer as to what privileges you are granted. While certain other states have legislation in place that encourages breast-feeding, currently none but the four states mentioned have laws mandating employer cooperation. This situation may change soon; there may even be new laws in place by the time you read this book. To know for sure, you can check with the Department of Labor in your state.

That said, under the Pregnancy Discrimination Act, you can initiate a lawsuit against your employer, suing for the right to stay home the entire time you are breast-feeding. Be advised, however, that it will likely be a long and costly endeavor. Several cases tried under this law have been decided in favor of the employer.

Experts say the best thing you can do is talk sensibly and openly to your boss, supplying as much information as possible concerning the ex-

Making the Big Announcement: What to Do

In order to make use of any of the legal protections afforded to you during pregnancy, you obviously have to inform your employer that you're pregnant. While many women choose to keep their pregnancy a secret until they begin to "show"—usually around the second trimester—doing this may not work to your advantage. That's because many of the pregnancy-related complaints apt to affect you at your job—such as morning sickness, fatigue, nausea, even temporary memory loss—are more likely to

tended health benefits (to mother and baby) of nursing as well as how these benefits can translate into fewer sick days and less downtime—and ultimately less lost revenue for the company.

And don't be surprised if a female boss seems less sensitive to your needs than a male boss, particularly if she did not nurse her own children or if she stopped when she returned to work. She may view your request for on-the-job nursing privileges as a judgment of her own parenting skills.

To keep this from happening, make certain that she understands that you view this as an entirely personal choice that may not be right for every woman but is something you personally need and desire. Ultimately, it may help if your doctor can write a short note explaining that nursing is important to you and your baby, and that the need to express milk on a regular schedule is important to the health of your breasts and to ensure that your milk continues in good supply. While presenting such a letter may prove extremely embarrassing for you—especially when employers are not legally bound to honor such requests—it could help you win the nursing privileges you desire.

If you do feel self-conscious about requesting breast-feeding privileges, please recognize that the nursing issue has received national attention and that thousands of women share your concerns. Also keep in mind that asking for these privileges does not in any way cast aspersions on your professional abilities nor make any statements about the importance of your job or your professional position.

occur during the first trimester. If your coworkers, or particularly your boss, don't know you are pregnant, they might just assume something a lot more debilitating is wrong with you. Perhaps even more important, if your job involves any factors that could potentially cause harm to you or your baby, the sooner you let your boss know you are pregnant, the sooner you can make the necessary changes—and ultimately the better off you and your baby will be.

All things considered, telling your immediate supervisor or your employer about your pregnancy early on is a smart move—and you should do so before informing any coworkers. And, say experts, you shouldn't let your news "slip out" as you pass your boss on the way to the watercooler. Instead, request a formal meeting to discuss an important issue—without giving any hint about your pregnancy.

HOW TO TELL YOUR BOSS YOU'RE PREGNANT

While the purpose of calling a meeting with your boss is, of course, to announce your pregnancy, experts from *Parenting* magazine say you also need to take this opportunity to show just how capable and prepared you are to continue your professional life. Come to the meeting prepared to answer a series of questions before your boss even asks. These can include:

- How long you intend to continue working during your pregnancy

- How much time off you will need after giving birth

- Whether you plan to return to your job full or part time

- Suggestions for how your work can be handled in your absence—who might take over for you while you're away, and whether your work can be reassigned to a staffer or if hiring a temp will be necessary

Also let your boss know if you will be available at home once you stop working and how much (or how little) the company can depend on your input while you are on leave. Experts say it's also a good idea to find out as much as you can about how your company handles maternity leave prior to this meeting. If there is a company handbook available, it will most likely discuss policy on maternity leave—so read it and become familiar with what may already be expected of you *before your meeting*. You can network with other women in your company who have already given birth and find out how your firm handled their leaves. If you belong to a workers union, now is the time to check on their maternity policies. Remember, you don't have to tell anyone you are pregnant while on your fact-finding missions.

Once the meeting with your boss or supervisor has concluded, follow up with a short, written memo that recaps your conversation. Your memo should state approximately when you expect to stop working, the length of your leave, how your work will get done in your absence, and your plans for returning after your baby is born. Keep a copy of the letter for your files, including the date it was submitted.

As soon as your boss is aware of your condition, you are free to tell coworkers—or to keep the good news private as long as you like. Do keep in mind, however, that each of your colleagues may have a totally individual reaction to your pregnancy, which may have nothing to do with you. Although for the most part having a baby is a deeply personal experience, ironically, it also can push the buttons of other people with whom you come in contact.

So be prepared for an assortment of reactions from colleagues— some will share your joy and enthusiasm, some may bitterly resent your condition, and some may even be emotionally upset by your pregnancy, particularly if they are having problems conceiving. The important thing, however, is that you don't allow yourself to be professionally intimidated by anyone's reaction to your pregnancy, whether a boss or a colleague.

Ten Tips for a Healthier Working Pregnancy

Regardless of whether you work to the very end of your pregnancy or stop at any point along the way, there are things you can do to make work easier and less stressful for you and your baby.

With the help of experts from the Workcare Group, a worksite health promotion organization in Charlottesville, Virginia, and doctors from the University of California at Irvine Department of Obstetrics and Gynecology, here are a few ideas to help blend your pregnancy with your career demands in a safe and healthy way.

#1: DON'T BE "SUPERWOMAN"

Get lots of rest when you aren't at work and reduce home chores as you get closer to your due date. Studies show that just one and a half hours of extra rest daily increases uterine blood flow and improves the supply of oxygen and other nutrients to your baby.

#2: RELAX WHEN POSSIBLE

If your job has a ladies' room or even a gym with floor mats, lie down on your left side for ten minutes during your lunch hour.

#3: LEAVE WORK EARLY WHENEVER YOU BEGIN TO FEEL EXHAUSTED

If you commute using public transportation, don't be afraid to mention that you are pregnant to the bus driver or train conductor and ask for assistance in ensuring you get a seat.

#4: TRY TO NEGOTIATE A FLEXIBLE WORK SCHEDULE

If you suffer from morning sickness, ask about coming in later and working later. If you get very tired in the late afternoon—particularly if you are a very early riser—ask to come in earlier and go home sooner.

#5: TELECOMMUTE WHENEVER POSSIBLE

Try to group assignments that require your presence at the workplace into two or three days and save up projects that you can do at home for one or two days of the week. Another alternative is to work part of the day at the office and part at home—but make certain to have a phone line that is always open for office contact.

#6: ASK FOR HELP

If any one job assignment or task is starting to overwhelm you, and particularly if you feel your health is beginning to suffer, talk to your boss about getting the help of another employee or even a temp worker to fill in the gaps. If need be, ask that the project be reassigned to someone else and take a different, less stressful assignment.

#7: SNACK

To keep energy levels high and to avoid nausea and heartburn, take a selection of snacks to work and eat something every few hours.

#8: PREPARE A PREGNANCY EMERGENCY KIT

Keep the kit in your desk drawer or work locker. It should include peppermint or lemon hard candies for nausea; an extra pair of undies and a sanitary napkin for incontinence accidents; an Evian Face Mister for instant cool-offs; and a cache of crackers, pretzels, or lemon wafer cookies for snacking.

#9: WRITE NOTES TO YOURSELF

To offset the "spaciness" and memory loss of first-trimester pregnancy, keep a small notebook handy at all times and write down important work reminders. Jot down *anything* you think is important for you to remember.

#10: DON'T BE A HEROINE

If you can, start your maternity leave a week or two before your due date to give yourself time to rest up for the big day.

A Final Word: When It's Time to Quit Your Job and When to Return to Work

If you are like many women, you'll probably have a good idea when it's time to stop working—either because your doctor has advised you to do so or simply because you are too exhausted to continue. There are, however, some specific recommendations you should be aware of—guidelines developed to help decrease the risk of pregnancy health concerns for you and your baby. According to the American Medical Association, if your job requires that you spend more than four hours a day on your feet, you should consider stopping work or switching to a desk job beginning in your twenty-fourth week of pregnancy. If your job requires you to spend more than thirty minutes out of every hour on your feet, consider shifting to more sedentary work tasks by week thirty-two.

Some medical experts also suggest that if your job requires rigorous and constant heavy lifting, climbing, pulling, pushing, or bending below the waist, you should stop work by week twenty. If these activities are considered moderate—meaning you don't do them all day long and you have sufficient rest periods—you can safely continue working until about the twenty-eighth week of your pregnancy. You should, however, consider stopping work soon after conception if you have a history of premature birth or miscarriage or if you are expecting twins, triplets, or quadruplets. Also consider cutting your work hours if you are diagnosed with gestational diabetes or high blood pressure.

Most important, listen to your doctor and take his or her recommendations concerning how long you should continue working, as well as the level of work you can safely perform during each of your trimesters. As you read earlier, there are laws in place that can help you to receive some kind of financial benefits should your health demand that you stop working earlier than anticipated, so don't ignore your doctor's warnings, no matter what your financial status.

You might also want to consider the distance from your job to your home or, more important, to your doctor's office or the hospital where you plan to deliver your baby. If you do commute long distances or if that commute is very long due to heavy traffic, this fact should also figure into your decision about when to stop working.

Regarding returning to work after your baby is born: Much of your decision may be mandated by how you feel and the health of your baby. Assuming you are both fine (and the vast majority of new mothers and new babies are!), then returning to work becomes strictly a personal choice. In a survey of some 1,300 new moms conducted by Parent-soup.com, a full two-thirds stayed away twelve weeks or less; one-third took less than eight weeks to get back to work.

But whether you take the full three months, less, or longer, remember that many of the same workday precautions apply as when you were pregnant:

- Avoid fatigue by napping whenever possible.

- Try to arrange to do some of your work at home.

- If possible, go back part time rather than full time until your body readjusts to your work schedule.

- Push for a flexible work timetable, coming in later and working later or starting earlier and leaving earlier, to accommodate your baby's needs.

- Try to arrange work hours to reduce time spent on the road commuting.

Above all, make certain that your spouse understands that it may take you a while to get back in the swing of a regular work routine at the same time you are still learning to be a new mom. Don't be afraid to enlist his help with household and baby chores.

Most important, if you find yourself overwhelmed, depressed, or fatigued, consider taking additional time off. Remember, you have twelve full weeks of family leave coming to you after childbirth, and you can split that up any way you like. If you do return to work after six weeks, but two months later find yourself in need of a break, you are entitled to take the second six weeks of your leave. But even if you feel better after some time off—and especially if you don't—make certain to see your doctor for a complete checkup before returning to work.

Is It Healthy,
Is It Harmful?

A Lifestyle Guide for the Mother-to-Be

- Is it safe to use a tanning bed?

- Can I paint the nursery while I'm pregnant?

- Is it okay to fly in my third trimester?

- Can I use a nicotine patch to quit smoking?

- Are computers still dangerous to use during pregnancy?

- What about anthrax vaccines, radiation exposure, West Nile virus—how will they affect my baby?

If you're like most women, these are just some of the worries and fears that can boggle your mind during pregnancy. You worry for your own health, certainly, but you worry about your baby most of all. But regardless of what you may read in the headlines, when it comes to pregnancy, there are actually relatively few things in today's world that should cause you worry or fear. According to research published in the journal

Seminars in Reproductive Medicine in 2000, there are, in fact, less than two dozen lifestyle factors or activities that have been proven harmful to pregnancy. The other side of the argument, of course, is that not every factor suspected of harming a pregnancy has been adequately studied. As a result, some experts contend that, at least in a few instances, we may not know enough about certain lifestyle factors—or what happens when two or more factors combine—to declare them safe.

That said, it's important to remember that there are *always* ways to reduce your risks and still live the life you want to lead. The best place to start? By learning a little something about the factors we do know matter, including which ones are relatively safe. Using this information, you can begin to assess your own personal risk profile and make common-sense changes that will benefit you and your baby the most.

Alcohol and Your Pregnancy: What You Should Know

Although scientists continue to discover many health benefits associated with moderate alcohol consumption, this is definitely not the case when it comes to pregnancy—a time when even small amounts of alcoholic beverages have the potential for causing major problems. One reason is because each time you take a drink, your baby "takes a drink" as well. While your grown-up body can metabolize that alcohol in just four to five hours, leaving your system clean, it can take your baby up to eighteen hours to accomplish the same thing. Because alcohol slows body functions, including heartbeat and breathing, it's not hard to see how even one drink can substantially reduce your baby's vital signs, affecting the intake of oxygen and other nutrients necessary for growth and development.

Should deprivation of vital nutrients continue for any significant length of time, your baby can develop fetal alcohol syndrome (FAS)—a group of serious physical, psychological, and behavioral birth defects that can last a lifetime. According to the March of Dimes, FAS is the leading cause of mental retardation, affecting some 12,000 U.S. babies each year.

Real Life

DRINKING BINGE AND MY PREGNANCY TEST

Q: My husband and I had been trying to get pregnant for nearly two years and had no luck. One night we had a horrible fight about this. He walked out and I was so devastated I started drinking . . . and kept on drinking for the whole night. Three days later I found I out I was four weeks pregnant. My husband and I made up—and I'm now in my third month of pregnancy, and haven't touched a drink since that night. But we're still both scared that my one-night binge damaged the baby I didn't know I was carrying. What are the chances that something did go wrong?

A: There is some good news in your story and some definite signs that things are okay. First, you have made it through the first twelve weeks without a problem—which means you are probably past the point where any alcohol you did consume could have caused a miscarriage. The second piece of good news is that you haven't had a drink since—meaning your baby was exposed to alcohol only that one time.

All things considered, experts say you probably have very little, if anything, to fear. While there remains no "safe" level of alcohol during pregnancy, even heavy drinking for one night or a few drinks occasionally before discovering you are pregnant does not put your baby at any dramatically increased risk of problems. Most often alcohol-related birth defects are confined to those women who drink *throughout* their pregnancy, not just once or twice.

To help ease your mind completely that your baby is okay, by week seventeen of your pregnancy your doctor can perform a simple, painless ultrasound exam and, if need be, a slightly more complicated test called an amniocentesis soon after that. Both tests can offer you and your husband reassuring news that your baby is most likely very healthy and was not affected by your one-time drinking experience.

HOW MUCH ALCOHOL IS TOO MUCH?

If you're thinking that perhaps only the babies of heavy drinkers are at risk, think again. The March of Dimes also reports that more than *50,000 babies* are born in the United States *each year* with some degree of damage, often the result of relatively small amounts of alcohol regularly consumed by their mothers during pregnancy. Often those damages fall under the heading of fetal alcohol effects (FAE)—a series of psychological and behavioral problems that can continue throughout your child's life.

In at least one study, researchers from the University of Washington in Seattle followed a group of children whose mothers reported having three drinks per day during their pregnancies. By age four, these children were scoring lower on basic intelligence tests. At ages seven and fourteen, all were having problems in school, often with math skills. Studies conducted by the March of Dimes on children with FAE from birth to age ten found that not only did they score lower on intelligence tests, they were also frequently diagnosed as hyperactive, nervous, and inattentive, with aggressive, even destructive behavior patterns.

More recently, in a study published in October 2002 in the journal *Alcoholism: Clinical and Experimental Research,* doctors from the University of Pittsburgh School of Medicine reported that consuming as little as one and a half drinks *per week* during pregnancy could have a negative impact on your baby. In their studies, babies were born smaller and weighed less, and had smaller heads—particularly when mothers drank during their first trimester. The research, which also followed some of these children up to age fourteen, found that as teens, they were still smaller and shorter than other kids their age.

"It's a clear sign that there is a long-term effect on these children . . . and it goes down to fairly low levels of exposure," reports study leader Nancy Day, an epidemiologist at the University of Pittsburgh.

For a small but significant number of pregnant women, the effects of drinking alcohol can have even more tragic results, increasing the risk of miscarriage, stillbirth, and early infant death. Indeed the more a womn drinks during pregnancy, and the earlier she starts, the greater those risks.

The bottom line: Both the American College of Obstetricians and Gynecologists and the March of Dimes join with physicians nationwide in advising pregnant women that *no* level of alcohol is considered safe to consume during pregnancy.

HOW ALCOHOL AFFECTS YOUR BABY

Amount of Alcohol per Day	How It Affects Your Baby
4 ounces or more	Induces fetal alcohol syndrome
2 to 3 ounces	Reduces birthweight
1.5 ounces	Causes deficits in IQ (5–7 point reduction)
5 drinks a night, once weekly	Memory problems and attention deficit

Source: *Seminars in Reproductive Medicine*, Vol. 18 (2000).

Smoking and Your Pregnancy:
What You Should Know

The message is clear: Smoking and pregnancy *don't* mix. But that's a fact that is frequently ignored. One reason is that nearly every woman who continues to smoke during her pregnancy does so because she knows at least one other woman who also smoked and her baby turned out just fine. Sometimes it may even have been your own mother who smoked or even drank during pregnancy, and you certainly turned out okay.

But it is precisely this Russian roulette effect that can make smoking so particularly dangerous—because you never really know when the wheel will spin in your direction, and your baby will be the one affected.

What can happen? According to the American Lung Association, when a mother smokes, the poisons she ingests—particularly carbon monoxide—make their way to the placenta, preventing the baby from receiving the nutrients necessary to grow and develop.

The end result:

· A decrease in birthweight by up to 30 percent

· An increased risk of premature delivery by up to 14 percent

- An increased risk of serious, placental-related complications that can threaten both your life and that of your baby

In addition, when you smoke during pregnancy, it increases your baby's *lifetime* risk of asthma and other breathing disorders. In studies published as early as 1995 in the *Journal of Family Practice Medicine,* doctors showed how babies of mothers who smoked during pregnancy were more likely to suffer learning disabilities. More recent studies have revealed how smoking can also increase your child's risk of birth defects, including cleft palate. What's more, the March of Dimes reports that, each year, more than 10,000 hospital admissions to neonatal intensive care units are due to parental smoking—which also causes up to 10 percent of all infant deaths. Smoke after your baby is born, and you increase their risk of dying from sudden infant death syndrome (SIDS).

PROTECTING YOUR BABY:
WHAT EVERY SMOKER CAN DO

While quitting smoking is clearly the best gift you can give your baby, even cutting down on the amount you smoke can have beneficial effects. If you quit even midway through your pregnancy, you can reduce your baby's risk of significant health problems. According to experts from the Centers for Disease Control, if you stop smoking early in your pregnancy, your risk of having a low-birthweight baby reverts to that of a woman who never smoked.

Even better news: Studies show that one of the most popular "quitting" aids—nicotine patches—is safe to use during pregnancy. In studies conducted at the State University of New York at Stony Brook, doctors found that, at the very least, the patches were no more dangerous than cigarettes, and appear to be far less hazardous in terms of baby's health. The patches, which deliver a continuous but low level of nicotine through your skin, are considered safe even during the third trimester, a time when many smoking-related complications occur. While other forms of nicotine replacement—gums or lozenges—were not tested, doctors say they have no reason to believe they wouldn't score a similar safety profile.

That said, it's also important that your nicotine replacement product supply *less* than what you would normally get from cigarettes—so how much you smoke must figure into your decision of what method you will use to quit. If you smoke only a few cigarettes a day, then that may turn out to be less harmful than even a low-dose patch. So, if you do decide to use a nicotine replacement product during pregnancy, make sure to talk it over with your doctor first. What's more, make certain that you **never** smoke when using any of these replacement products. Doing so can dramatically increase your baby's—and your own—health risks.

Pregnancy and Real Life: What's Healthy, What's Not

From house-cleaning chemicals to paint fumes, mosquito repellent to fertilizer, swimming pools to tanning beds, perhaps nothing gets our attention more than headlines that tout the untold dangers of the lifestyle activities we pursue every day. And while there is no shortage of scary stories in the news, in many instances exposures must be extensive and occur for long periods of time before they cause any real harm. In other instances, there are things you can do to immediately make even questionable factors safe and less threatening to you and your baby.

To help you do just that, the following guide addresses some of the most commonly asked questions concerning pregnancy and lifestyle matters—queries submitted by pregnant women of all ages, from all walks of life, and living in all parts of the United States.

Answers are based on the latest medical studies and the opinions of experts from the American College of Obstetricians and Gynecologists, the March of Dimes, the National Academy of Sciences Institute of Medicine, and the Centers for Disease Control, along with Harvard environmental expert Jennifer R. Gardella, R.N.C., and Kaiser Permanente's Dr. De-Kun Li. Together these resources offer you the background information you need to open a dialogue with your own doctor and determine which lifestyle factors are most important to you and your baby.

To help you locate the information you need quickly and easily, the subjects of these questions are arranged in alphabetical order. Position in the list does not in any way indicate a level of importance or concern.

Your Healthy Pregnancy Lifestyle Guide

AIR TRAVEL

Q: I have to make several business trips that are scheduled for what will be my twenty-eighth and thirty-second weeks of pregnancy, and again at thirty-five weeks—and I have to fly to get there. Is air travel safe in the third trimester—or anytime during pregnancy?

A: According to guidelines released by the American College of Obstetricians and Gynecologists in December 2001, as long as you are suffering no pregnancy complications—like high blood pressure, placental abnormalities, or history of premature labor or miscarriage—and you are in good cardiovascular health, you can safely fly domestically up to your thirty-sixth week of pregnancy, and up to your thirty-fifth week for international flights.

Do be aware, however, that most airlines have some restrictions about flying in the third trimester—with many requiring a doctor's letter of permission signed no more than forty-eight hours before you plan to travel. Since ticket agents aren't likely to mention this, you need to ask about each airline's specific policies. For more flying comfort, request a roomier bulkhead seat, on the aisle. This can make it easier for you to get up to walk around during the flight, which is important for your circulation, and easier for you to get to the rest room, too.

Since dehydration is always a problem when flying, whether you are pregnant or not, drink plenty of water before, during, and after your trip. Experts also suggest that you wear support stockings on long flights and periodically move your legs about. Doing both will help reduce the risk of blood clot formation in your lower legs. And, of course, always wear your seat belt, strapped low on your hipbone between your abdomen and your pelvis. For extra protection, carry a copy of some personal medical information, including your blood type, any history of health problems, and a list of all medications you are currently taking, as well as any drug allergies. Include your doctor's name and phone number and your due date. Finally, before leaving on your trip, ask your doctor for a referral to a physician at your destination.

CELL PHONES, BEEPERS, AND PREGNANCY SAFETY

Q: I use a cell phone all the time, and now that I'm pregnant I'm wondering if it's safe. I'm also concerned because I live relatively close to a cell phone power station. Is that going to cause me any harm?

A: The issue with cell phones focuses on nonionizing radiation. Known as RF waves, they are emitted from the phones during use and from the cell towers that send the phones their signals. According to Robert Brent, M.D., Ph.D.—a member of the Health-Physics Society and an expert in this area—the level of nonionizing radiation generated by these phones is extremely small and is very different from the kinds of ionizing radiation exposure that we do know is harmful. As a result, he says, cell phones give us little to fear. "This type of exposure does not put your fetus at risk for a measurable increased risk of birth defects," says Dr. Brent.

In addition, John Molder, professor of radiation oncology at the Medical College of Wisconsin, says cell phone base stations are safe as well. "There is no laboratory or epidemiological evidence at all that RF radiation at the power levels associated with public exposure from mobile phone base station antennas is associated with miscarriages or birth defects," he says.

While most studies agree with both these experts, at least one report—a study of some 6,000 baby chicks released by doctors from the University of Bastide in France—found that those exposed to cell phones and towers were five times more likely to die. At least theoretically, some doctors concluded that heavy cell phone use *may* be causing some women to lose their babies before they even know they are pregnant.

Perhaps more important, studies published in the journal *Epidemiology* in 2002 suggest that while single items like cell phones may not cause much harm during pregnancy, when combined with other sources of nonionizing radiation, such as microwaves or computers, they could represent a small but significant threat. Until these studies are either verified or refuted, err on the side of caution by never carrying your cell phone near your stomach—particularly if it is on—and limit use to necessary calls only during your pregnancy.

COLOR TVS, MICROWAVES, COMPUTERS, ELECTRIC BLANKETS, AND MISCARRIAGE

Q: I love snuggling under an electric blanket and using a heating pad on my back when I sit and read. Now that I'm pregnant, my husband says the electromagnetic fields from these appliances and from my computer can harm my baby. Is he right—or just being a nervous daddy?

A: Father may know best. According to the latest research, there may be some new cause for concern. Generally speaking, electromagnetic fields are energy waves that surround many electric devices—heating pads and electric blankets, color TVs, microwave ovens, computers, and most office equipment. These energy waves are measured in milligauss (mG). The number of mGs an appliance is emitting determines whether it has the potential to harm your pregnancy.

In the latest research, published in the journal *Epidemiology* in 2002, investigators from Kaiser Permanente's Division of Research in Oakland, California, found that women exposed to higher-than-normal levels of mGs during their first ten weeks of pregnancy were six times more likely to miscarry. Those at greatest risk, says researcher Dr. De-Kun Li, were women with a history of pregnancy loss or fertility problems.

The study, which involved 969 women, is considered particularly important because each wore a special meter designed to measure hourly mG exposure over a twenty-four-hour period—giving researchers a good idea of the level of exposure during an average day.

The end result: The scientists discovered that as little as 16 mGs a day are enough to harm a pregnancy. By comparison, standing next to your microwave oven while you heat up a cup of coffee can expose you to anywhere from 100 to 300 mGs. However, walk just three feet away while it's on, and exposure drops to insignificant levels.

Although study results need to be replicated before doctors can say for certain that these devices cause any clear-cut pregnancy risks, based on the current research, many experts suggest limiting exposure and avoiding those products used close to or on your body—such as a heating pad or electric blanket. Stay at least three feet away from your microwave, color TV, computer, and any other office or home machines you use every day, and you should be safe.

DRY-CLEANING CHEMICALS AND PREGNANCY FEARS

Q: My husband is a dry-cleaning freak—he takes all his clothes to the dry cleaners' and insists that in between I use the home dry-cleaning kits in our dryer. He's also obsessed with spot cleaners, which he uses on his clothes and our carpets. I can't stand the smell, and now that I'm pregnant I'm wondering if I should even be exposed. Is there any information on the dangers of these chemicals?

A: Hubby may have to learn to live with a few spots and stains—at least until your baby is born. Research shows that exposure to at least some of the chemicals used in the dry-cleaning process can cause adverse reproductive outcomes in animals and humans. This is particularly true of chemical solvents such as perchloroethylene, toluene, xylene, and stylene, often found in dry-cleaning compounds. While truly dangerous exposures usually occur only in an occupational environment—where you would use these chemicals all day long—at least theoretically, the continued exposure you describe could hold the potential for problems.

To reduce risks, ask hubby to remove the plastic from newly cleaned clothes and air them out *before* hanging them in your bedroom closet. If you do use a home dry-cleaning kit in your dryer, toss the clothes in and leave the room—don't hang around folding laundry while fumes are in the air. When the clothes are done, don't open the dryer until it's cooled down. Then let clothes air in a well-ventilated room before you put them away. Better still, have hubby take care of his own at-home dry cleaning. It's also probably not a good idea for him to use any products containing solvents to clean clothing, furniture, or rugs while you are pregnant unless you remain out of the house until all vapors disappear.

HOME REPAIR AND PREGNANCY RISKS

Q: I'm an avid do-it-yourselfer and was just about to start stripping and revarnishing my living room floors when I found out I was pregnant. My mom says all home repairs are off limits now, especially varnishing. How dangerous is it, particularly if I use a water-based paint product?

A: In general, paint companies and those that manufacture wood stripping products, glues, adhesives, or almost any item used in home repair have not invested much time or money in testing the health effects of their products when used during pregnancy. Some medical studies, however, have shown that certain ingredients found in some home decorating products can increase the risk of miscarriage. At least one study, published in the *Journal of the American Medical Association* in 1999, found that regular exposure to organic solvents found in many paint and restoration formulas resulted in an increased risk of severe physical birth defects. Again, the most dramatic are going to coincide with regular, daily use of these ingredients—in a work environment, for example—with far fewer problems anticipated with short-term or one-time use.

Still, experts say there are some ingredients you should completely avoid during pregnancy. They include ethylene glycol, ethers, lead, mercury, and formaldehyde-releasing biocides, at least some of which can be found in paint and some glues. You should also stay away from most paint thinners, such as turpentine. In addition, avoid spray paints, since their formulation can make it easier to inhale any potentially toxic fumes. According to experts from Harvard Medical School and Beth Israel Deaconess Medical Center, oil-based paints and paint thinners generally contain more potentially harmful chemicals than water-based or latex paints, but you should observe at least some precautions when working with either one, including keeping windows open and cross-ventilation going while you work.

As to the varnishing, putting it off until baby is born is probably the best idea. If you find you must do it yourself, wear gloves, a mask, and protective clothing, and don't take any food or drink into the room while you work.

MARIJUANA, COCAINE, AND PREGNANCY RISKS

Q: I enjoy smoking marijuana occasionally since it helps me relax. My husband says it's very bad to use during pregnancy, but I'm too embarrassed to ask my doctor if he's right. Can smoking marijuana hurt my baby?

A: Because few women will admit to using drugs during pregnancy, there are few studies documenting the dangers. In the studies that have been published, however, regular use of marijuana has been shown to increase the risk of low birthweight. When combined with either cigarettes or alcohol—a common combination—doctors say health problems associated with all three can be greatly exacerbated.

But marijuana is not alone in its potential to harm your baby. According to experts from the American College of Obstetricians and Gynecologists, heroin and other narcotics can cause preterm birth and fetal death, while cocaine and crack can cause birth defects or even fetal death. Hallucinogenic drugs like PCP and LSD have been linked to birth defects, including neurological damage. Depending on the drug used during pregnancy, and the amount, babies can be born addicted and suffer dangerous withdrawal symptoms after birth.

But it's not just your baby who's at risk. When you use certain drugs during pregnancy, you also increase your risk of high blood pressure and stroke. Cocaine use can cause your placenta to detach from your uterus, increasing your risk of hemorrhage, preterm birth, and fetal death. The bottom line here: If it's wise to avoid even helpful medications during pregnancy, it's a no-brainer to realize that social drugs should be off your list as well.

PESTICIDES AND LAWN CHEMICALS

Q: You can't walk down a street in my town or even visit a neighbor without being exposed to bug sprays and weed killers—pesticides of all kinds. I'm concerned that spending any time out of doors, even on my own lawn, is going to harm my baby, but my husband says I'm just worrying for nothing. Also, he wants to continue to have our regular exterminator visits while I am pregnant—they spray for roaches. Is this safe?

A: Certainly at least some of your fears are justified since, in general, most experts advise pregnant women to avoid pesticide exposure as much as possible. While there is little evidence that low-level exposure is harmful—such as walking down the street where pesticides have been used on a lawn—some studies suggest that, in higher doses, at least some of these products may cause birth defects. What's more, University of South Florida chemical expert Professor Richard Pressinger says we should be concerned about what we *don't* know—for example, how low levels of these substances react when they are combined with other factors that can be harmful, such as cigarette smoke, alcohol, or even other chemicals.

That said, you should not be fearful of spending time out of doors, or even attending a barbecue or a wedding where the lawn was recently sprayed. In most instances, infrequent low-level exposures, particularly out of doors, are not likely to affect you or your baby. However, you should try to avoid direct contact with pesticides. According to experts from the March of Dimes, you might consider skipping the exterminator visits during pregnancy and instead use non–odor-emitting bait stations to protect against infestation. If spraying must be done, stay out of your house twice as long as the product recommends—up to three days in some instances. Also, clear away all food, dishes, and utensils, and afterward ask someone else to wash countertops or furniture that may have been exposed to the spray.

Experts from the March of Dimes suggest that you never apply weed killers, fertilizers, or pesticides yourself, either indoors, on plants and flowers, or outdoors on your lawn. If others are using these chemicals in your yard, or anywhere close to your home—like a neighbor's yard—close all your windows and doors and shut off air-conditioning until the work is completed. When gardening, always wear protective gloves, and thoroughly wash your hands afterward. Also be sure to wash all fruits or vegetables that come from your garden, or anywhere that pesticides may have been used.

SWIMMING POOLS AND CHLORINE EXPOSURE

Q: I love to swim, and my doctor says it's a great prenatal workout. But I just read an article that claims chlorine exposure is dangerous during pregnancy and could cause miscarriage. I don't live near a lake or ocean, and a pool is the only place where I can swim. Is this warning justified?

A: It's true that swimming is an excellent prenatal workout, and in most instances the chlorine presents few, if any, risks. In fact, to date, only one study—research published in the journal *Occupational and Environmental Medicine* in April 2002—found a problem. These researchers documented that pregnant women who regularly swam in public pools appeared to have an increased risk of miscarriage, while those who did give birth had babies at greater risk for low birthweight or neurological defects.

As far as the researchers could determine, the problems were likely linked to the potentially carcinogenic by-products found in chlorine—the chemical used to keep pool water, as well as drinking and bathing water, clean. Other studies have shown that exposure to at least one potentially harmful by-product of chlorine—chloroform—was 141 times higher during a one-hour swim than during a ten-minute shower in chlorinated water. Clearly, the amount of chlorine found in most pools is far higher than that found in your home water supply. And because chlorine can be absorbed through the skin, it's clear that your risks would be greater during a one-hour swim than during a ten-minute shower.

As to whether or not swimming holds any real danger for your baby, the answer is "not likely." In fact, in order for the studies to have true meaning, the findings would have to be duplicated many times over, and with large groups of women—and so far that has not happened. The bottom line: If you are at high risk for miscarriage, you may want to avoid swimming in a pool during your first trimester, when potential damage would be greatest. What can also help: Seeking out a small public pool—like the kind found in a high school—since, generally, the fewer people who use it, the less chemicals needed to keep pool water clean. While chemicals used in private home pools may be easiest to control, unless it's your own, you don't really know how well the water is being monitored. If you do have a home pool, consider hiring a professional tester to check for excessive chlorine. Also, follow directions on all pool chemicals and remember, more is *not* better; use only as much as is needed to keep water pure and clean, and you and your baby should be safe.

In addition, you may want to switch to nonchlorinated natural spring water to use for drinking and cooking during pregnancy. While there are no studies to show this is any safer, at least theoretically it will reduce your risk of chlorine exposure even further.

TANNING BEDS/SELF-TANNERS

Q: I am a very pale-skinned redhead, and I love the way my skin looks when I use a self-tanner. I'll be hitting my sixth month of pregnancy when summer rolls around, and I need to know if it's safe to use these products late in pregnancy. If not, are tanning beds any safer? I'm trying to avoid the sun.

A: Staying out of the sun is a smart idea, particularly during pregnancy. Not only can sun exposure increase your risk of skin cancer, during pregnancy it also increases your risk of melasma, or pregnancy mask, as well as other skin discolorations. What you may not realize, however, is that the same risks apply when you use a tanning bed. Although many salons boast that you are getting only the "safer" UVA rays and not the burning UVB rays, there may be little comfort in those claims.

According to New York University dermatologist Dr. Darrell Rigel, in natural sunlight 90 percent of the burning rays are UVB and only about 10 percent are UVA. But once you switch to tanning in a salon, the power of the UVA rays jumps 300 to 500 times over what you get from the sun. The bottom line, he says, is that you won't get a tan without damaging your skin, and in the end it doesn't matter which rays do the damage; the risk of skin cancer is the same. You should also know that melasma, or pregnancy mask, can be caused by either UVA or UVB rays.

As to self-tanners, so far there appear to be no medical or government reports citing problems when used during pregnancy. Since the active ingredients stay on top of your skin and aren't absorbed into your bloodstream, most doctors agree they are safe. However, from strictly a cosmetic standpoint, if you happen to experience even slight pregnancy skin discolorations such as pregnancy mask, the self-tanner could make the problem appear darker and more obvious. Also remember that self-tanners are not protection from the sun, so you'll still need a sunscreen.

WEST NILE VIRUS, MOSQUITO REPELLENT, AND MISCARRIAGE

Q: I'm three months pregnant and it's August in Connecticut—which is mosquito heaven! I was already scared of catching West Nile virus before, and now a friend told me that pregnant women are virtual mosquito magnets. Is this true, and if I do catch West Nile, is that the end of my pregnancy?

A: Since mosquitoes are generally attracted by warm body temperatures, and your temperature during pregnancy is generally higher than normal, it is true that you may attract more mosquitoes than usual. It doesn't mean, however, that you'll be calling swarms of those buggers from all cities and towns. What it does mean is that you probably should avoid being outdoors during dawn and dusk, when most mosquitoes are out. If you do go out, wear light-colored clothing that covers as much of your body as possible—a long-sleeve shirt, for example, with long pants and socks.

In regard to your fear of West Nile virus, according to the Centers for Disease Control (CDC), the risk of a pregnant woman becoming severely ill from a single mosquito bite is very remote. Even if the mosquito is infected with West Nile, fewer than 1 percent of people bitten and infected become severely ill, whether they are pregnant or not. And CDC experts also confirm that West Nile virus is not particularly threatening to a pregnancy, over and above whatever symptoms the disease normally causes.

Once your baby is born, however, a new risk profile for West Nile virus may come into play. In October 2002, Michigan state health officials confirmed that a newborn had contracted West Nile virus from breast milk. Although the mother developed the infection after receiving a tainted blood transfusion during her delivery, at least theoretically the same thing could have happened if she had contracted the virus via a mosquito bite. The woman nursed her baby for two weeks before she herself was diagnosed with the disease, and the baby was diagnosed shortly thereafter. Both reportedly recovered within a few weeks.

Early symptoms of West Nile virus include headache, low-grade fever, slight body aches and pains, and sometimes a skin rash and swollen lymph glands. More severe symptoms include the onset of high fever and a brain inflammation known as encephalitis—which occurs mostly in adults over age fifty.

When it comes to protecting against mosquito bites, there comes another word of caution, this time about the popular repellent ingredient known as DEET. According to the Children's Health Environmental Coalition, a Canadian advocacy group, DEET *can* cross the placenta—which means it can get into your baby's bloodstream. Environmental researchers Eugene Pergament, M.D., Ph.D., and Amy Stein Rissman, M.S., from the Illinois Department of Public Health, believe there is at least some cause for concern over the use of DEET during pregnancy, particularly during the first trimester. If you do use a repellent containing DEET, the recommendation is to use it sparingly, and purchase those formulations containing the lowest concentration—no more than 30 percent. Products in this category include Fite Bite 30 Insect Repellent Spray (30 percent); Green Head Fly, Insect and Tick Repellent (30 percent); Buggspray—Vanilla Scent (25 percent); Off! Deep Woods (24 percent); Repel: Family Formula Aerosol (15 percent); and Cutter All Family Insect Repellent (7 percent). In early pregnancy use of any DEET-containing products should be limited to only when absolutely necessary. What is reportedly safe to use, however, are the sonic repellents—the tiny electronic devices that give off a high frequency sound wave that reportedly insects just can't stand. You won't hear the frequency, however, and neither will your baby.

X RAYS

Q: My sister is pregnant and broke her leg. The doctor gave her several X rays even though he knew she was pregnant. Isn't this harmful to her baby?

A: Radiation comes in many forms—the most common of which is ionizing radiation, the kind associated with an X ray. Although ionizing radiation has been proven to cause birth defects and other pregnancy problems, for the most part this occurs only when you are exposed to large doses or small, regular doses over a long period of time. According to the American College of Radiology, no single diagnostic X-ray procedure carries enough radiation to cause a woman or her baby any harm.

Certainly it's a good idea to avoid any unnecessary exposure during pregnancy. And with the advent of ultrasound imaging as well as magnetic resonance imaging (MRI), many women can avoid an X-ray procedure. But when that's not possible, as in your sister's case, there is little to fear. What is a good idea, however, is to make certain that your radiologist—the person taking the X ray—knows that you are pregnant. Often you will be given some extra protection, such as covering your stomach with a lead apron, and making certain to avoid this area of your body as much as possible when positioning the X-ray equipment.

In case you're wondering about airport security radiation—currently, passengers only go through metal detectors, which do not emit any radiation. Only baggage is exposed to X rays, and the rays are well housed so that exposure is not a threat to anyone in the immediate vicinity.

Pregnancy and Life in the Twenty-first Century

Since the events of September 11, 2001, life—and pregnancy—will never be the same. Threats and concerns that we never could imagine are now stark realities we must face. And while it's important to keep our fears in the proper perspective, the knowledge of what to do if an emergency situation does arise can go a long way in helping to keep your pregnancy calm and serene.

For this reason, this chapter includes some general precautionary guidelines about some concerns that have made their way into the headlines. Remember, this information is not meant to frighten or disturb you, but rather to inform you and, it is hoped, ease your mind about having a baby in the twenty-first century.

ANTHRAX AND PREGNANCY: THE FACTS

As you may already know, anthrax is an extremely harmful bacteria that, as the terror mail scares of 2001 and 2002 have shown us, can be used as a biological weapon. Anthrax spores invade the body either through inhalation or a cut in the skin, with serious or even deadly results.

But in the event that anthrax exposure becomes a potential threat, the American College of Obstetricians and Gynecologists and the Centers for Disease Control advise that during pregnancy it is safe to take the recommended treatment—the antibiotic ciprofloxacin—for the recommended sixty days. It is also safe to be vaccinated against anthrax during pregnancy. In medical studies on over 4,000 female army recruits published in the *Journal of the American Medical Association* in March 2002, doctors reported *no* adverse effects when pregnant women received the vaccine. It also did not affect future fertility.

The anthrax vaccine was licensed by the Food and Drug Administration for use in humans in 1970. Prior to 1990, use was limited to those at highest risk, including certain veterinarians and laboratory workers. Since 1998 the U.S. military has given over 2 million doses of the vaccine to over 500,000 men and women without major ill effects. In the event that anthrax does become a threat during your pregnancy, talk to your doctor. He or she will undoubtedly have the very latest recommendations on prevention and treatment.

SMALLPOX AND PREGNANCY: THE FACTS

Although virtually all threat of the virus known as smallpox had disappeared from the world in the last century, in 2002 fears of infection surfaced once again. As a result of world tensions and the threat of terror attacks, the idea of a smallpox vaccine, not used in the United States since the 1970s, once again became a topic of discussion.

While getting an inoculation against this disease may become mandatory once again, right now vaccinations are considered voluntary, and pregnant women are not being advised to take part in the protection plan. The current recommendation by the U.S. Centers for Disease Control indicates that unless directly exposed to the smallpox virus, pregnant women should *not* get this vaccine—nor should anyone who lives with a pregnant woman and maintains what the government calls "household contact." This would include your mate and your children.

Smallpox is a potentially deadly virus for which there is no known treatment. The last case worldwide occurred in Somalia in 1977. Should you be exposed to the virus, or if the threat of exposure becomes exceedingly high, contact your obstetrician immediately for the latest advisories on protection and care.

NUCLEAR RADIATION AND PREGNANCY: THE FACTS

As bioterrorism fears became a reality, concerns over the safety of our nation's nuclear power plants also came to light. The most publicized fears concerned potential attacks on the facilities that ultimately could expose large surrounding areas to doses of potentially deadly radiation. If this should occur, nationwide health plans include the distribution of potassium iodide (iodine)—a mineral that can help deter the risk of developing thyroid cancer, one of the main consequences of radiation exposure.

The important news here is that an iodine pill is safe to take during pregnancy—in fact, iodine is a mineral necessary to your baby's development. While under normal conditions and with a normal diet you most likely get all the iodine you need, in the event of a nuclear accident, you will need this pill. Currently the Food and Drug Administration says that pregnant women exposed to a nuclear event can safely take 130 milligrams of potassium iodide in a one-time dose, in pill or capsule form, which will protect you and your baby.

Although this supplement is widely available without a prescription, never use this treatment without your doctor's express consent. If it becomes necessary to use potassium iodide during your pregnancy, your doctor will have the latest information on the dosages and forms that would benefit you and your baby the most.

Pregnancy and Your Lifestyle: A Final Word

While the rate of pregnancy catastrophes can be linked to whatever threat is looming during a specific decade or even century, it's important to remember that even under the most adverse circumstances, the vast majority of babies are born healthy and strong.

Certainly, for those who do suffer problems, even seemingly small effects can be a devastating blow to family and loved ones. But it's important to put the threat of problems in the proper perspective and realize that the odds are on your side for a healthy and happy pregnancy. In fact, most doctors now agree that stress, worry, and fear are far more likely to cause you problems than all the lifestyle threats put together—and, thankfully, these are factors you *can* control.

So when fears start to mount, simply turn off the evening news, stop reading that daily paper, and take time out to relax, and think happy, positive thoughts about having a healthy baby. In studies presented at the annual meeting of the Society of Behavioral Medicine in 2002, researchers from the State University of New York at Stony Brook reported that women who remained optimistic about their ability to control their pregnancy actually *did* control important birth outcomes. For the women who held positive thoughts about the outcome of their pregnancy, doctors saw a *reduced risk* of premature birth and low-birthweight babies. Even when the researchers controlled for the effects of diet, smoking, history of miscarriage, diabetes, or even stress itself, they found that the women who were positive thinkers had, overall, a more positive pregnancy outcome.

So, live a little, laugh a little, love a little, and worry less, and have a happy, healthy baby!

Year-Round
Pregnancy Care

Solutions for Your Everyday
Health Problems

You catch a cold; you're exposed to the flu; you go out to dinner and come home with stomach cramps; your cat allergy is flaring. Under normal circumstances, you'd probably know *exactly* what to do. But now you're pregnant and wondering if your symptoms are cause for alarm? Will your tried-and-true treatments work as well as they did before? Are they even safe to use?

If these are the kinds of questions running through *your* mind, you're not alone. Obstetricians report that most women don't know what to expect when even the most common ailments occur during pregnancy. And if you also happen to suffer with any chronic health concerns, such as asthma or migraine headaches, you may be at even greater loss over what to do during pregnancy.

The important thing to remember, however, is that there are effective and *safe* ways to deal with virtually any health problem you encounter without harming your baby. One key is, of course, to stay in close contact with your doctor and let him or her know whatever symptoms you are experiencing—certainly before you use any over-the-counter treatments or even pre-pregnancy prescription drugs.

But equally important is having some firsthand knowledge of what you can expect—how symptoms of even the most common ailments might differ during pregnancy, and what your available treatment options are. With this information in hand, you will be better prepared to work with your healthcare provider and take care of yourself to ensure that you sail through any temporary health setbacks with ease.

The Five Most Common Health Problems: What Every Pregnant Woman Should Know

PROBLEM #1: ALLERGIES

It could be sneezing, coughing, itching, a runny nose, watery eyes, or all of the above. The problem is allergies, and whether it's a seasonal event related to grass, trees, and pollen or a year-round condition caused by foods, pets, or pollution, if you had allergies prior to getting pregnant, you're going to have them now.

And don't be surprised if you develop a nasal allergy for the first time during pregnancy, particularly a stuffy or runny nose that can last all three trimesters. Pregnancy hormones can cause even women with little or no previous allergy problems to develop considerable nasal congestion during this time. Or they can aggravate an existing allergy, so that symptoms worsen during pregnancy.

Your Pregnancy Medicine Chest: Treating Allergies

Whenever possible, your first line of defense should always be to avoid allergic triggers. If that's not possible, or if despite your best efforts you are still experiencing symptoms, then medication may become necessary. If so, there are some safe options for you to try. Remember, however, that while some allergy drugs have been shown to be safe for use during pregnancy, data on others may be less clear. That's why it's important that you always consult with your allergist as well as your obstetrician before de-

An Expert's Opinion on

YOUR PREGNANCY WARDROBE AND ALLERGIES

Can what you wear increase your allergic reactions to other factors, such as cat dander or dust mites? The answer is yes—at least according to a group of Australian researchers.

In their study, published in the *Journal of Allergy and Clinical Immunology* in December 2000, wearing a wool sweater appears to increase exposure to dust mites ten times more than garments made of fabrics such as cotton or a synthetic blend. Exposure to cat dander was eleven times greater in those wearing wool compared to other fabrics. The researchers say the best garments to wear to decrease allergic reactions are those made from freshly washed cotton knits like the kind used to make T-shirts. They proved to harbor the fewest allergens.

If you're allergic to cat dander, what you wear can make a difference even if you think you won't be in an environment where cats are present. The study also showed that cat dander can be found on the clothes of non–cat owners after they simply had social or business contact with people who do own cats, even when the cats themselves were not present. The particles, they explain, spread from the cat owners' clothes to the clothes of others, particularly to those who wear wool or other loosely woven fabrics. Here again, the answer is to wear cotton, or cotton/polyester knit fabrics, which reduce transmission of the dander particles.

ciding what to use. Getting their advice is even more significant today than in the past, since so many prescription allergy drugs are now available over-the-counter.

To help you work with your doctor on finding the right medication for you, the American Academy of Asthma, Allergy and Immunology (AAAAI) offers the following information on some of the most commonly used treatments:

Real Life

ALLERGY SHOTS AND PREGNANCY: WHAT TO DO

Q: I was in the process of taking allergy shots when I found out I was pregnant. Now I'm wondering if it's safe to continue, or if I should stop until after my baby is born. I really have terrible allergies and shots are a tremendous help. What can I do?

A: According to the American Academy of Asthma, Allergy, and Immunology, there are no known adverse effects from taking allergy shots during pregnancy. Experts agree, however, that you need to inform your allergist that you are pregnant and also tell your obstetrician that you are taking allergy shots. It is hoped that the two doctors can confer and make certain that the treatment you are receiving is best for you and your baby. If you do continue with the shots, one or both physicians should carefully monitor your dosage and your reactions. If you have never had allergy shots before, experts say pregnancy is *not* the time to begin treatment. Wait until after baby is born.

Allergy Drugs Considered Safest to Use

Antihistamines like chlorpheniramine (Chlor-Trimeton) and diphenhydramine (Benadryl) are both considered safe—they don't cross the placenta, so they won't affect your baby. They can, however, cause you to feel drowsy and possibly experience some motor impairment, so keep this in mind if you have to drive. While nonsedating antihistamines are available, according to the AAAAI, they've not been properly evaluated for use in pregnancy.

Allergy Drugs You Can Consider Using

Claritin and cetirizine (Zyrtec). Although both lack a significant track record, doctors say that so far they appear to cause no problems during pregnancy. Additionally, the few studies that have been done have offered encouraging results. You can also talk to your doctor about nasal sprays containing the active ingredient oxymetazoline (Afrin, Neo-Synephrine).

While there are no precise safety studies on this drug, it is only minimally absorbed into the bloodstream, so it may be an option to consider. Anti-inflammatory nasal sprays (Nasalcrom and Becoran) are another alternative, but AAAAI experts say only if symptoms persist *and* worsen over the course of several days. While there are some newer anti-inflammatory nasal sprays on the market, there is little or no data on use in pregnancy. That said, because they are also minimally absorbed, many doctors say they are probably safe as well.

Allergy Drugs You Should Avoid

Most decongestants, particularly pseudoephedrine (Sudafed), should be avoided. Studies published as early as 1992 and as recently as 2001 have shown that this drug may increase the risk of a serious gastrointestinal defect in your baby. Experts from Beth Israel Deaconess Hospital and Harvard Medical School in Boston caution that you should avoid virtually *all* over-the-counter allergy medications containing epinephrine during pregnancy.

ALLERGY RED ALERTS

· *Never* take an allergy medication prescribed for you prior to pregnancy without talking to your doctor first.

· Don't use any over-the-counter allergy products without your doctor's okay.

· If you are seeing an allergist, make certain he or she knows you are pregnant, and be sure to tell your obstetrician if you are under the care of an allergist.

PROBLEM #2: THE COMMON COLD

As you may have already discovered, *nothing* is common during pregnancy. Sometimes even a simple cold can leave you feeling more stuffy, as well as achier and crankier than you ever remember feeling. One reason is that high estrogen levels can cause mucous membranes to dry out and swell. This, in turn, can make the congestion from a cold seem much worse. And as your pregnancy progresses and your uterus grows, your baby will push harder against your diaphragm. This not only reduces your lung capacity, making it harder to breathe, it can also make even mild infections seem much worse.

But it's not only that you might *feel* more sick; you may actually be a little more ill than usual. Experts from the University of Michigan Health System report that because during pregnancy your immune system is somewhat compromised—operating at less than optimal levels—even a simple cold can dig in its heels and make you feel a lot more miserable for a lot longer.

Your Pregnancy Medicine Chest: Treating a Cold

Most experts agree that the best treatment for a common cold is bed rest and lots of fluids, including chicken soup, which may be among your best pregnancy remedies. Not only is this a great comfort food, there is some real science behind the cure. In a study published in 2001 in the journal *Chest,* doctors documented that chicken soup stopped the movement of immune system cells to the site of inflammation—which in turn helps reduce symptoms like coughing and sneezing.

Another natural treatment option is hot tea with honey, which is particularly good for a sore throat. The steam from the hot liquid will help decrease your congestion, while the tea can act as a mild anti-inflammatory. Studies have also shown that honey has mild antiseptic qualities and could help control the local growth of bacteria.

Still another favorite is the saltwater gargle—¼ teaspoon of salt to about 8 ounces of warm water. It may stop the pain of your sore throat almost immediately. The reason: The saltwater solution mimics fluids found naturally in the body, so it can provide comfort to irritated tissues.

If you just can't *live* without *something* in a medicine bottle for that hacking cough or chest congestion, talk to your doctor about over-the-counter products like Robitussin, Robitussin-DM, and Vicks cough syrup. Acetaminophen (Tylenol) is reportedly best for aches and pains and low-grade fever, but don't take it without your doctor's okay.

COMMON COLD RED ALERTS

- Always talk to your doctor before trying any over-the-counter or prescription drugs while you are pregnant.

- If your cold produces green or yellow nasal mucus, or if it lasts more than seven days, call your doctor. You could have sinusitis, a bacterial infection that does require antibiotics.

- If you are running a fever with your cold, call your doctor right away—even if other symptoms seem mild. (For more information on coping with fever in pregnancy, see the next section.)

PROBLEM #3: THE FLU

While pregnancy doesn't increase your susceptibility to the flu, if you manage to catch this virus while pregnant, you are up to five times more likely to develop serious complications, including pneumonia or bronchitis. Thus, it's imperative that you avoid contact with anyone who has the flu and also situations where flu germs can be easily spread, such as crowded elevators, buses, trains, or even department stores. This is particularly important between December and March, when flu season is peaking.

According to the Centers for Disease Control (CDC), the best way to avoid nearly all risk is to have a flu shot. This, they say, is a must if you are going to be more than thirteen weeks' pregnant during flu season. While most doctors recommend that you get your vaccine sometime after your first trimester, if you are considered a high risk for flu complications—if you have asthma, heart disease, or diabetes, for example—CDC experts say the protection this vaccine provides is so vital, it's okay to get your shot *anytime*, even during your first trimester. Since it takes several weeks before flu shots become fully effective, the optimal time for a vaccine is between October and November.

YOUR PREGNANCY MEDICINE CHEST: TREATING THE FLU

If you do contract the flu, you can safely try all of the natural remedies used to treat a cold. But when it comes to using more traditional medications, most obstetricians say to avoid them. First, all strains of the flu are caused by a virus, so general antibiotics won't help you. More important, the antiviral flu medications that became available as early as the 1980s have not yet been tested adequately on pregnant women. So they are not considered safe to use.

If, however, you are running a temperature of 101 degrees or more, medications to control fever will be necessary. That's because studies show that high fever during pregnancy can increase your baby's risk of neural tube defects, life-threatening malformations of the brain or spine. Other studies have shown a small but significant increased risk of heart or abdominal wall problems as well if Mom's temperature rises too high. In addition, sustaining a temperature of 102 degrees or more during early pregnancy could dramatically increase your risk of miscarriage.

According to the March of Dimes, if your doctor approves, acetaminophen (Tylenol) can be your best fever remedy. The usual dosage is two regular-strength tablets every four hours—but again, check with your obstetrician or midwife first.

What can also help: Making certain that you don't skip your prenatal vitamin while you are sick. A study of some 2,000 pregnancies conducted by Dr. Lorenzo Botto from the National Center on Birth Defects and Developmental Disabilities in England found that women who took a multivitamin high in folic acid during pregnancy reduced their baby's risk of birth defects, even if they ran a fever while pregnant.

Finally, doctors say that a cool compress on your forehead can help reduce fever and make you feel more comfortable, as can drinking plenty of cool fluids, particularly water. Do not, under any circumstances, attempt to "sweat down" your fever with hot drinks or hot showers.

FLU RED ALERTS

· Don't get a flu shot if you are allergic to eggs.

· Don't get a flu shot unless you get your physician's okay.

· Contact your doctor immediately if you run a fever of 101 degrees or more.

PROBLEM #4: DIARRHEA, NAUSEA, AND VOMITING

No matter what the cause, a queasy, upset stomach, with or without vomiting, can seem like a pregnancy nightmare. But as bad as you may feel at that moment, most mild gastrointestinal upsets are not dangerous to Mom or baby. Most of the time, say doctors, they resolve on their own, usually within forty-eight hours, even if you don't take any medication.

There are, however, times when diarrhea and nausea *can* be symptoms of something much more serious for pregnant women: food poisoning. Although most foodborne illnesses are relatively mild, changes in your metabolism and your circulation during pregnancy mean that even a small amount of bacteria in your food can cause major stomach upset. So you are likely to feel a lot worse than friends or family who may have contracted the same bug.

What's more, several bacteria linked to food poisoning, including *Listeria monocytogenes,* salmonella, and *Escherichia coli* (*E. coli*), can have some devastating effects on your pregnancy. (See Chapter 6.) Thus, if you believe your upset stomach may be food related, contact your doctor right away. You may need a round of antibiotics to help reduce the risk of problems for you and your baby.

So, how do you know if you have food poisoning or just a simple stomach virus?

Stomach Virus: Symptoms are usually limited to cramps, diarrhea, and perhaps nausea and vomiting; they normally peak within twelve to twenty-four hours and then usually begin to wane.

Food Poisoning: Symptoms usually start out like the flu, with fever, chills, a headache, and that sore-all-over feeling; this is *followed* by a quick progression to nausea, vomiting, and diarrhea. In addition, food poisoning often causes severe abdominal cramping—much worse than anything you may have experienced before with a simple stomach virus.

Your Pregnancy Medicine Chest:
Treating Diarrhea, Nausea, and Vomiting

Among the biggest threats, even with simple diarrhea, is the risk of dehydration. Thus, the most important treatment is to increase fluid intake as much as possible. If water makes your stomach feel worse, try tea, ginger ale, or clear soup broth.

Experts from the American College of Obstetricians and Gynecologists frequently recommend the BRATT diet: short for bananas, rice, applesauce, toast, and tea to help control vomiting and diarrhea, as well as replace some of the vital nutrients you may have lost.

Since most obstetricians suggest you stay away from as many medications as possible during pregnancy, don't be surprised if your doctor does not prescribe an antidiarrheal unless your symptoms become severe or last longer than forty-eight hours. That said, in the event you do need medication, research shows that some are considered safe to take during pregnancy. These include drugs like Donnagel and Kaopectate, neither of which is absorbed by the body—so they never reach your baby. A third medication known as Loperamide (Imodium) has not been tested in pregnant women, but studies on animals reveal it is likely safe to use as well.

The one diarrheal medicine you might want to avoid during pregnancy is Pepto-Bismol or any drug containing the active ingredient bismuth subsalicylate. Although occasional use may not prove harmful, animal studies have shown that salicylate, which is related to bismuth subsalicylate, may increase the risk of birth defects.

If your nausea is related to an upset stomach, then the queasy feeling should go away soon after your diarrhea or other gastrointestinal upsets clear. To speed things along, most doctors recommend natural remedies, such as sucking on crushed ice or sipping an icy cold ginger ale. A cup of chamomile tea can also settle your stomach and quell nauseous feelings at the same time. And don't forget you can try any of the remedies for morning sickness explored in Chapter 1.

If, however, queasiness persists more than twenty-four to forty-eight hours, talk to your doctor about whether anti-nausea medications used for morning sickness can help. These include antihistamines, such as the allergy medication Benadryl (diphenhydramine) or the classic seasickness remedy known as Dramamine (dimenhydrinate). Although both are considered safe to use during pregnancy, never take any anti-nausea drug without first discussing it with your doctor—even if he or she has prescribed this medication for you in the past. Continued nausea or vomiting that is not related to morning sickness may need specific medical attention.

GASTROINTESTINAL RED ALERTS

· **Don't take any antidiarrheal medications until you check with your doctor.**

· **If diarrhea or vomiting continues for more than thirty-six hours, call your doctor.**

· **Phone your doctor** *immediately* **if:**

   · **cramps are severe;**

   · **diarrhea or vomit contains blood;**

   · **you exhibit any of the signs of food poisoning, including fever, chills, and other flulike symptoms.**

PROBLEM #5: MIGRAINE HEADACHES

For most women a simple headache, usually caused by tension, is somewhat self-limiting. Often it goes away on its own within a few hours or less. But for those who suffer with migraine headaches, pain, plus nausea and vision problems, can continue for days—and often medication is required to ease symptoms. If you've never had a migraine, don't be surprised if you get your first one during pregnancy. The American Council on Headache Education reports that up to 15 percent of migraines occur for the first time during pregnancy.

But even if you have had these headaches in the past, there is unfortunately no real way of knowing how you will be affected during pregnancy. While many women report fewer headaches after conception, others say they saw no change during pregnancy. Still others confirm more severe headaches after they become pregnant.

If your migraines are normally hormone dependent—usually occurring at a certain point in your menstrual cycle—you may be in for more frequent headaches during your first trimester, a time when hormone levels are a little erratic, much the way they can be just prior to the onset of each monthly menstrual cycle. As levels stabilize later in pregnancy, you are likely to have far fewer headaches, or even none at all. Another comforting thought: Although a pregnancy migraine can make *you* feel awful, studies show these headaches aren't harmful to your baby and *won't* increase the risk of birth defects or other developmental problems.

What's also important to note, however, is that because both estrogen and progesterone levels drop sharply right after giving birth, you may be at risk for a migraine *after* delivering your baby, or within the first week after childbirth. The good news here is that often these headaches are far less severe than the typical migraine.

Your Pregnancy Medicine Chest: Treating Headaches

Most experts agree that, if possible, migraine medications should be discontinued during pregnancy, particularly during the first trimester—mostly because there is only limited safety data available on use during this time. That said, if your symptoms are severe, there are a number of medications that have been shown to be relatively safe—if you use them in moderation and under the watchful eye of your doctor.

According to the American Council on Headache Education, these include pain medications such as acetaminophen (Tylenol) and the narcotics Percocet or Vicodin, and, as migraine prevention treatments, certain beta blockers (high blood pressure drugs) and antidepressants. If nausea and vomiting are significant, drugs such as Emetrol and Tigan are considered safe to use during pregnancy.

In addition, the American Medical Association's Migraine Center cautions against using either aspirin or medications known as NSAIDs—nonsteroidal anti-inflammatory drugs such as Motrin (ibuprofen) and Naprosyn or Aleve (naproxen). These medications have been linked to an increased risk of gastrointestinal bleeding and, say experts, may also interfere with the labor process.

When it comes to popular migraine-specific medications—drugs known as triptans (sumatriptan, noratriptan, zolmitriptan), as well as er-

An Expert's Opinion on

COPING WITH PREGNANCY
HEADACHES NATURALLY

While you may be used to popping a pill to cope with a migraine, headache expert Dr. Dawn A. Marcus says there *is* a better way. Known as flare management techniques, these simple head and neck movements can help break the cycle of muscle tension linked to headache pain and ultimately help you control your migraines. According to Dr. Marcus, the following exercises might help get you through the night.

Oscillatory Movements
This exercise involves rhythmically turning your head, from a center starting point, to the side, away from your pain, and back again, at the rate of about one move per second for a total of thirty seconds. Your turns should be gentle and no wider than 25 percent of your total range of motion. Rest for thirty seconds, and repeat exercise for thirty more seconds, or until pain decreases. Then switch sides, turning from the center point toward the side where pain is located. Rest, then repeat movements as needed, until pain begins to subside.

Positional Distraction
In this exercise, you place a one- to two-inch stack of books on the floor and cover them with a towel. Lying on the floor on your back, rest your head on the books so that their edge touches the center of your scalp, with your neck area free. Relax into the position, allowing your head to move up freely from your neck.

Important: If you are beyond your twentieth week of pregnancy, make certain that you don't lie on your back for more than five minutes. As with any exercise, check with your doctor before trying these flare management techniques.

gotamine or dihydroergotamine—it's important to note that long-term safety profiles have not been established. And while that lack of data has led the Food and Drug Administration to classify these medications as contraindicated for use in pregnancy, doctors say they can sometimes be helpful if taken in moderation and in conjunction with careful monitoring by a physician.

MIGRAINE RED ALERTS

· Never use a migraine drug prescribed prior to pregnancy until you check with your doctor first.

· If you are experiencing what you think is your first migraine, run your symptoms by your doctor—and don't try any over-the-counter remedies without your physician's okay.

· Try natural relief methods first, including lying down in a cool, dark room with as little noise as possible.

Asthma and Your Pregnancy: What You Need to Know

Among the most common chronic illnesses is asthma, a type of allergic response that causes a constriction in the airways and can make breathing extremely difficult. Affecting up to 7 percent of all pregnant women, when uncontrolled and untreated asthma can threaten not only a mother's life but also that of her baby. That's because your baby's total oxygen supply comes from your blood, so anything that affects your ability to breathe automatically affects your baby. When the oxygen supply is low, even for a short time, your baby can experience impaired growth. If oxygen deprivation becomes extreme, it will be difficult for the baby to survive.

According to the American Lung Association, uncontrolled asthma can also increase the risk of giving birth to a premature, low-birthweight baby, as well as increase your baby's risk of birth defects. The largest study ever on pregnancy asthma—research conducted by the Robert Wood Johnson School of Medicine in New Jersey in 1998—found it can also increase your risk of high blood pressure and preeclampsia as well as a number of labor complications.

While asthma symptoms may increase late in your second and early in your third trimesters, fortunately these problems are likely to decrease during the last four weeks of pregnancy—a time when your baby moves farther down in your uterus. This change of position relieves some pressure from your diaphragm, making breathing easier.

Even more important, as long as your asthma is under good control, pregnancy is not likely to increase your symptoms or make you feel worse. According to the American College of Asthma, Allergy and Immunology (ACAAI), up to two-thirds of pregnant asthma patients either see no change in symptoms or report they actually feel *better* during pregnancy.

If, by chance, your asthma does worsen temporarily, ACAAI experts say the most severe problems are likely to occur between the twenty-fourth and thirty-sixth week of pregnancy—after which time they usually subside. Even more good news: Studies show that nine out of ten pregnant asthma patients will sail through labor and delivery without experiencing any breathing problems.

MANAGING YOUR PREGNANCY ASTHMA: WHAT TO DO

Experts say your first line of defense should always be to modify lifestyle factors linked to symptoms. You should scrupulously avoid asthma triggers such as cigarette smoke, and maintain control over your environment, including using air filters to reduce exposure to dust and dander whenever possible. Also consider a flu vaccine after your third month of pregnancy, since respiratory infections can increase your risk of asthma symptoms.

If your asthma *does* require treatment, medication should be used sparingly and, of course, only under your doctor's supervision. Often the most important aspect of dealing with asthma during pregnancy is balancing the risk of treatment against the risk of no treatment.

When, however, medication is required, inhalers are often recommended. While they are not 100 percent problem free, studies have demonstrated that the benefits associated with most inhaled medications far outweigh any potential risks. Experts from the AAAAI report that because most inhaled drugs produce only a localized effect—with very little of the medication getting into the bloodstream—they are considered relatively safe for baby. Drugs in this category include Aerobid, Beclovent,

Real Life

THE SEX OF YOUR BABY AND YOUR ASTHMA

Q: I just found out I am carrying a baby girl. Since I have asthma, my aunt told me that I can expect to have a lot more attacks in my second trimester, because baby girls cause more problems than baby boys. Is my aunt off her rocker, or is this true?

A: Auntie *might* know best; it *is* possible that your child's gender may affect the severity of your asthma. In a study of thirty-four pregnant women published in the *British Medical Journal* in 1998, a group of London doctors found that of the eighteen women who were carrying boys, only four reported a worsening of asthma symptoms, while eight reported an improvement. By contrast, of the sixteen women carrying girls, half reported asthma symptoms worsened with pregnancy, and none reported any improvement.

The study was limited to the first trimester, however, a time when many women experience the least number of asthma events. Thus, it's possible that as these pregnancies progressed, the odds may have changed in favor of girls. No matter what the sex of your baby, keep a close watch on symptoms, and do what you can to reduce asthma triggers. If problems occur, work with your doctor to find the medications that are safest for you.

Pulmicort, and Vanceril, and anti-inflammatory drugs such as cromolyn sodium, all of which help open blocked airways.

According to reports presented at the 2001 annual National Conference of Nurse Practitioners, you can also feel safe using most bronchodilator medications, such as albuterol, metaproterenol, pirbuterol, and terbutaline. As long as they are used properly—on an emergency basis for immediate help in breathing—they are considered safe. Newer asthma medications—drugs like Singulair (montelukast), Accolate (zafirlukast), and Zyflo (zileuton)—are simply too new to chart safety concerns, so experts warn they should be used judiciously and with extreme caution during pregnancy.

The class of asthma medications known as methylxanthines (theophylline) are prescribed less often to pregnant women due to neonatal withdrawal symptoms, which can occur if these drugs are used throughout the pregnancy. Studies show that babies born to mothers who regularly used these medications while pregnant were jittery, irritable, and demonstrated heart rhythm problems.

Most important: *Don't use any asthma treatments without checking with your doctor first, even if you think the medication is safe.* Since every pregnancy is different, only your personal physician can determine which asthma drugs are right for you and your baby.

Sex, Infection, and Conception: Important Warnings

Although it may seem as if the words "pregnancy" and "sexually transmitted disease (STD)" don't belong in the same sentence, the unfortunate truth is that they do. Studies show that each year thousands of pregnant women require treatment for an STD—due either to the recurrence of a previously contracted infection or to one contracted for the first time during pregnancy. Even if you are in a totally monogamous relationship, it's possible that one or both of you could be harboring a "silent" infection—a disease that may suddenly flare up during pregnancy.

While all STDs should eventually be treated, there is some debate over whether some might be better left alone until after baby is born. Note, however, that certain infections—including genital herpes and gonorrhea—can be passed to your baby during delivery, and your newborn can suffer some devastating health consequences. For this reason always bring to your doctor's attention any V zone symptom you feel is out of the ordinary—discharge, odor, blister, itch, or pain—and discuss any need for further testing and treatment. While not all drugs routinely used to treat STDs are safe during pregnancy, in many instances there are medications that can help.

If an active genital herpes infection is present near your due date, discuss the option of cesarean section with your doctor. Delivery this way can reduce virtually all risk of passing the infection to your baby.

Childhood Diseases and Your Pregnancy: What You Can Catch from the Children in Your Life

Whether you are a teacher, day care worker, or mother, or spend time around friends or family who have children, whenever there are youngsters present there is a risk of childhood diseases. While most of these infections don't pose any real harm to adults, that situation can change if you contract them during pregnancy—a time when some otherwise minor illnesses can have some devastating effects.

To help you understand more about your risks and what to do if exposure occurs, check out the following guidelines. Prepared with the help of the Organization of Teratology Information Services, the American Academy of Family Physicians, and the March of Dimes, these suggestions will help you learn what to do to avoid illness and what can help if you do get sick.

CHICKEN POX

Symptoms: Spread by droplets of infected respiratory fluids that make it into the air or by direct skin contact with an infected person, the hallmark of chicken pox is an itchy, red blistery rash that spreads over the body within about five days. Soon after, the tiny blisters break and dry scabs result. Direct exposure to the virus within your own household increases your risk to about 90 percent.

What You Should Know: According to the March of Dimes, 7 out of every 10,000 pregnant women contract chicken pox, a disease caused by the varicella virus. While most go on to have healthy, normal babies, up to 2 percent are born with birth defects, including eye problems, underdevelopment of limbs, small head size, and developmental delays. If you are exposed to chicken pox, call your doctor right away. Prompt treatment, including an injection of a preparation known as VZIG (varicella-zoster immune globulin), may reduce *your* risk of serious complications, including pneumonia. It is not known whether VZIG also confers protection to your baby.

While there are no medications to treat chicken pox—the virus runs its course and burns out in about ten days—you should be monitored closely during this time, making certain to control fever. Doing so can reduce additional health threats to your baby. Once the virus clears, and you are past the seventeenth week of pregnancy, ultrasound exams can help ensure that your baby has not suffered any ill effects.

Important to note: If you had chicken pox in the past, you are immune to this virus. What's more, you can also obtain a varicella vaccine, which is considered safe if administered up to three months *prior* to when you conceive. You should not, however, be vaccinated after you are pregnant.

RUBELLA (GERMAN MEASLES)

Symptoms: A flat, red rash that usually lasts about three days and often is accompanied by swollen glands, joint pain, and a low-grade fever.

What You Should Know: Rubella is a mild illness when contracted during childhood, but it can hold grave and serious complications for your baby if *you* contract this virus during pregnancy. According to the March of Dimes, about 25 percent of babies born to mothers who contract rubella in their first trimester—particularly during the first eleven weeks of pregnancy—are born with congenital rubella syndrome, a group of birth defects that includes vision disorders or blindness, hearing defects, heart abnormalities, mental retardation, and sometimes developmental delays and movement disorders. Fortunately, infections contracted after twenty weeks of pregnancy are much less likely to result in any problems.

Although there is a rubella vaccine, it is not safe to administer during pregnancy. Because rubella can have such devastating consequences, many doctors now recommend that all women get vaccinated three months prior to when they plan to get pregnant. Since many pregnancies are unplanned, however, this prevention strategy doesn't always work.

If you had rubella as a child or if you were vaccinated in the past, you are immune now. If you aren't certain, a simple blood test can give you the answer; so do ask your doctor about this test. If you do contract rubella, there is no treatment, other than bed rest, fluids, and controlling fever. Unless you know for certain that you are immune, any exposure to this virus should be reported to your doctor right away.

THE FIFTH DISEASE

Symptoms: Caused by parvovirus B19, it is called "the fifth" disease because it was the fifth in the list of the most common causes of childhood rash and fever. And, in children, the primary symptoms are a distinctive, red slapped-cheek rash, fever, and sometimes headache, sore throat, and joint pain. In adults, the rash is less likely to appear, but joint pain and swelling along with flulike feelings are common.

What You Need to Know: Roughly half of all adults are susceptible to this virus, including pregnant women. While it won't increase your baby's risk of birth defects, it can cause him or her to develop anemia—a condition represented by a low red blood cell count. If your baby's anemia is severe, life-threatening complications may develop. While sometimes the problem clears on its own, when it doesn't your baby may require a blood transfusion while still in the womb. In addition, when contracted early in pregnancy, the fifth disease can dramatically increase the risk of miscarriage. If you are exposed to this virus, call your doctor right away.

While there is no drug treatment available, it's important that your baby's health is monitored during this period. Ultrasound exams are your best tool for ensuring that your baby is fine. In certain instances, your doctor may suggest a procedure called PUBS—percutaneous umbilical blood sampling—to test baby's blood for signs of anemia.

CYTOMEGALOVIRUS (CMV)

Symptoms: While children can harbor this disease with few if any symptoms, some adults can develop a mononucleosis-type illness, with sore throat, fatigue, low-grade fever, and body aches. Unlike a cold, it does not generally cause a runny nose and sneezing, and unlike the flu, it does not normally cause a high fever.

What You Need to Know: Far and away the most common viral infection in adults and children, cytomegalovirus can be passed via saliva, urine, blood, or mucus, or it can be transmitted sexually. Many adults contract CMV while caring for small children, particularly when changing diapers. If contracted during pregnancy, there is up to a 40 percent chance that you will pass CMV to your baby. According to studies published in the journal *Obstetrics and Gynecology* in 1999, this is much more likely to occur in your third trimester—a time when you should be extra wary of contracting CMV. Indeed, each year some 40,000 U.S. babies are born with this virus, with up to 8,000 affected with learning difficulties, vision or hearing loss, or other neurological defects. About 800 babies a year die from an active CMV infection present at birth. If you are exposed to CMV, tell your doctor immediately. While there is no treatment available right now, several drugs look very promising. In addition, a number of tests are available to help ensure that your baby has not suffered any damage.

Note: Among the best ways to prevent CMV infection is to wash your hands frequently whenever you are in contact with young children or any adults who may be infected. Carefully dispose of any soiled diapers or tissues, and avoid sharing drinking glasses and eating utensils with small children—even your own, particularly if they are in day care. Studies show that up to 70 percent of children between the ages of one and three may be excreting this virus.

Medication, Self-Care, and Pregnancy Safety: What You Should Know

If you have ever questioned the safety of a medication prescribed to you during pregnancy, it's a sure bet that your doctor or pharmacist relied on a letter identification system created by the Food and Drug Administration to ease your mind. That coding system uses the letters A, B, C, D, and X to classify the safety profiles of medications when they are prescribed during pregnancy. And it works well to alert us to the two dozen

Real Life

Head Lice, Kindergarten, and Pregnancy

Q: I was baby-sitting my seven-year-old niece for a week, and during that time she came home from school with a case of head lice. By the time I found out what was wrong, I had them too. I'm nearly three months pregnant and worried about using the medicated shampoos that the doctors recommend. Are they safe, and are there any alternative treatments?

A: Because there is little data on pregnancy and the safety of these medicated shampoos, rinses, and lotions, many doctors don't feel comfortable recommending them, particularly during the first trimester. The next best treatment is to remove the lice by hand—and it's not as daunting a task as it may seem. First, purchase a lice comb from the drugstore; it's a comb with extremely fine, thin teeth. Working with small sections of hair, insert the comb as close to your scalp as possible and slowly pull it through to the ends of your hair. If you spot any of the pearly white nits—lice eggs—pull them out with your hand or the comb. Dip the comb in a bowl of warm soapy water, rinse, and repeat on each section of hair several times. Flush whatever you pull from your hair down the toilet. You will probably have to repeat this procedure every few days for a week or more.

In addition, a group of Harvard researchers has found that olive oil is an extremely effective way to kill head lice—and give your hair a deep conditioning treatment at the same time! The oil works by smothering the lice eggs, keeping them from breathing. To use this treatment, coat sections of your hair with small amounts of olive oil and use the lice comb to pull it through—coating and combing several times for each strand. Let the final oil treatment set for five to ten minutes, then shampoo with very hot water, followed by a blow-dry on high heat. Repeat this treatment every few days until all the lice are gone.

If you haven't already done so, you should also wash all your linens and clothes, and anything your niece touched, in very hot, soapy water, then place them in a dryer turned on high. Clothes that can't be washed or dry cleaned should be sealed in a plastic bag for two weeks. Be cer-

or so drugs that form category X—those proven to cause harm when used during pregnancy.

As important as the FDA coding system is, new research has begun to reveal it may have some alarming flaws. One such study, published in the journal *Obstetrics and Gynecology* in September 2002, proved just how little we know about many of the most commonly prescribed medications for pregnant women. More specifically, researchers revealed that of the 468 drugs approved by the FDA between 1980 and 2000, risks related to pregnancy remain undetermined in a whopping 91.2 percent—even though most of the drugs were between fifteen and twenty years old at the time of the study. Even more disturbing, say study authors, is that many of the drugs commonly prescribed for pregnant women—such as Zithromax, Biaxin, Claritin, and Ambien—lack *any* sort of documentation regarding safety of use during pregnancy.

At least part of the problem is that it is unethical to include pregnant women in drug trials, so it can take years before doctors amass enough personal experience to know which medications are safe to use. But another problem, say experts, is that once a drug is approved for sale, the FDA does not require manufacturers to perform *any* additional clinical studies or even active surveillance for the risk of birth defects. While some manufacturers voluntarily set up these registries, often it can take years or even decades before any solid data is available.

Yet experience has taught us something—and, as you have discovered in this chapter, doctors *do* feel confident about recommending a number of medications. So, do trust in your doctor's judgment if he or she decides a treatment can help you. At the same time, you can help your doctor and your baby by not insisting on having medication each time you don't feel well during your pregnancy.

You can also help protect your health while avoiding excess medications, if you pay attention to the following three simple rules. Endorsed by both the American College of Obstetricians and Gynecologists and the American Academy of Family Physicians, they can help ensure that medication use is safe and appropriate during your pregnancy.

1. **Never** take any medication from friends or relatives, even if their symptoms are similar to yours and they took the drug during

FDA DRUG CLASSIFICATIONS

Category A: Controlled studies in women failed to demonstrate risks during the first trimester; no evidence of risks later in pregnancy; the possibility of causing fetal harm is considered remote.

Category B: Either animal studies have shown no fetal risks, with no studies in women, or animal studies showed an adverse effect during pregnancy, but these findings were not confirmed in women during the first trimester. There is no data on these drugs when used later in pregnancy.

Category C: Either animal studies have shown adverse effects in the fetus, with no studies in women, or studies in women or animals are not available, making risks undetermined. According to the FDA, medications in this category should be used only if the potential benefit to the mother outweighs all risks to the baby.

Category D: There is positive evidence of human fetal risk, but certain benefits might make these risks acceptable—for example, if the mother's life depended on the use of this drug.

Category X: Studies in animals or humans have shown fetal abnormalities, or there is evidence of fetal risk in humans, or both. The FDA states that the risks of drugs in this category clearly outweigh any benefits. Not only are drugs in this category contraindicated for use in pregnancy, doctors are advised to refrain from prescribing these medications to any woman who *might* become pregnant while taking them.

Source: Food and Drug Administration

their pregnancy. Remember, every woman and every pregnancy is unique; medications are generally not safe to pass from woman to woman.

2. **Never** increase the dosage or frequency of a prescription or over-the-counter medication without checking with your doctor first. Often the safety of drugs is determined by the amount that's used—so never dismiss your doctor's recommendations.

3. **Always remember** that all drug regimens should be as short as possible during pregnancy. When your doctor says it's time to stop taking a medication, heed that advice and stop. At the same time, don't stop taking any drug unless your doctor tells you to—particularly antibiotics, which generally require a full course of treatment for a complete cure. If your symptoms continue after your finish your medication, don't refill a prescription without checking with your doctor first.

Herbs and Your Pregnancy Safety

If you're like most women, you probably believe that natural, alternative treatments are far healthier than traditional medicines during pregnancy. But according to Dr. Jan Friedman, medical director of the March of Dimes, "natural does *not* always mean safe." In the case of herbal supplements, Dr. Friedman cautions that "natural really means unregulated."

Since few safety studies have been conducted on the use of herbs in pregnancy, many of the supplements you might otherwise consider safe have at least the potential to cause you or your baby harm. To help you quickly spot the products you should avoid, the March of Dimes offers the following lists of herbs and combination supplement formulas that, for one reason or another, you should avoid during pregnancy.

Single Herbs to Avoid During Pregnancy

- Aloe
- Autumn crocus
- Black cohosh root
- Buckthorn bark
- Buckthorn berry
- Cascara Sagrada bark
- Chaste tree fruit
- Cinchona bark
- Cinnamon bark
- Colt's foot leaf
- Comfrey herb, leaf, and root
- Echinacea purpurea herb (injectable form)
- Fennel oil and seed
- Gingerroot (in large doses)
- Indian snakeroot
- Juniper berry
- Kava-Kava
- Licorice root
- Mayapple root and resin
- Parsley herb and root
- Petasites root
- Rhubarb root
- Sage leaf
- Senna leaf
- Uva-Ursi leaf

Herbal Combinations to Avoid During Pregnancy

The following combinations include both supplements and teas and should be avoided in any potency or form.

- Angelica root, gentian root, and fennel seed
- Anise oil, fennel oil, and caraway oil
- Anise oil, fennel oil, licorice root, and thyme
- Anise seed, fennel seed, and caraway seed
- Anise seed, ivy leaf, fennel seed, and licorice root
- Anise seed, marshmallow root, eucalyptus oil, and licorice root

- Caraway oil and fennel oil

- Caraway oil or seed, fennel oil or seed, with or without chamomile flower

- Licorice root, peppermint leaf, and German chamomile flower

- Licorice root, primrose root, marshmallow root, and anise seed

- Marshmallow root, fennel seed, Iceland moss, and thyme

- Marshmallow root, primrose root, licorice root, and thyme oil

Also consider avoiding all products that combine peppermint oil or leaf with any of the following ingredients: fennel oil or seed; caraway and/or fennel oil or seed with or without chamomile; senna leaf and caraway oil.

Currently the National Institutes of Health's National Center for Complementary and Alternative Medicine is studying the safety and effectiveness of many common herbal preparations, including those pregnant women often turn to for relief. To keep abreast of the latest findings, visit their website at www.NCCM.gov. Or contact the March of Dimes Resource Center at 888-MODIMES or e-mail them at: Resourcecen ter@modimes.org.

Pregnancy and Your Chronic Health Concerns: Some Special Advice

In the not-too-distant past, women with chronic health concerns were frequently told not to get pregnant. Even when health problems like diabetes or asthma were under good control, motherhood was discouraged. Fortunately, this situation is no longer true. While any chronic health concern will place you in the high-risk category, with proper care you *can* go on to have a healthy, happy, and successful pregnancy. Today even women with severe diseases, such as lupus, or those who have received a kidney transplant, can get pregnant and have a healthy baby.

While you may have to pay a bit more attention to even seemingly unimportant symptoms—things that other pregnant women may routinely ignore—you should be able to handle most pregnancy problems that come your way. Be aware, however, that some medications you may have relied on before to control symptoms or ease pain may not be safe to use during pregnancy—or you may have to use less of them. But with the help and support of your doctor and a little careful listening to your own body, pregnancy is possible—and a healthy pregnancy is a dream almost every woman can now achieve.

After the Glow

What to Expect After Your Baby Is Born

The hours, days, and weeks after you give birth are called the postpartum period. It's a time when you will not only get used to being a new mom, but also a time when your body will go through some major changes, including not only an adjustment in your shape and size, but also a dramatic shift in your hormones. While some of these changes you will no doubt welcome—losing your tummy and seeing your toes again—others may seem less than pleasant for a while. What can help: knowing what to expect and realizing that much of what you are experiencing is a normal part of your postpartum recuperation.

To help you do just that, what follows is the Afterglow Recovery Guide. Here you will find an overview of what you can expect during the three key phases of your postpartum period: the first six hours, six days, and six weeks after giving birth. Prepared with the help of the American College of Obstetricians and Gynecologists, the Nemours Foundation of Medical Centers, and some of the nation's top obstetricians, the information will not only help you better understand your postpartum recovery but also aid you in communicating with your doctor during this important time.

In addition, don't forget that many of the pampering tips you learned earlier work even better *after* you give birth, so don't be stingy with self-care time. Try to steal as least thirty minutes a week for yourself. Doing so can go a long way in helping you cope *and* feel more comfortable in the days and weeks following delivery.

Also remember that because every pregnancy is different and every recovery period somewhat unique, your postpartum timetable may not go exactly according to plan. You may respond faster or take longer getting through the various stages. So listen to your body, and don't hesitate to contact your doctor to check on any aspect of your health that may need attention during this time.

Your Afterglow Recovery Guide

THE FIRST SIX HOURS: WHAT YOU NEED TO KNOW

Whether you experienced a natural vaginal birth or a C-section delivery, expect to feel exhausted when it's all through! Just *how* tired you are will depend a lot on how long or difficult your labor was, whether you needed pain medication (it can make you feel sleepy afterward), and your overall physical condition both before and during your pregnancy.

If all goes well with your vaginal delivery, approximately thirty minutes after giving birth, your placenta separates from the wall of your uterus and is passed through your vagina. (If you had a C-section, the doctor removes the placenta during the surgery.) When this occurs, you will likely pass a significant amount of blood. Not to worry; this is normal. However, expect a nurse to be checking your urine output and monitoring your bleeding frequently during the first hour following delivery—this is also a normal part of labor recovery.

Although you may feel hungry after giving birth, don't be surprised if all you are allowed are ice chips and water. Should you require an additional medical procedure—to control bleeding, for example—having an empty stomach is to your advantage. Within an hour or so, you should be able to eat anything you like, so this is a good time to send a family member to the cafeteria for a snack. Or, better still, pack some après birth snacks in your labor/delivery bag—quick-energy, high-protein bars or a high-complex carbohydrate treat like oatmeal cookies or a whole-wheat bagel with jelly.

YOUR BODY: WHAT TO EXPECT

Within the next few hours, you will begin having a discharge of mucus, blood and tissue known as lochia. This can involve significant blood loss and the passing of large blood clots, particularly in the first eight to twelve hours following delivery. This is considered normal.

Because the area between your vagina and rectum was stretched dramatically during delivery, and may even have been torn, you're likely to feel some pain. If you received an episiotomy—a surgical cut in the perineum to aid in delivery—then you will definitely feel some discomfort in the hours following delivery. Your doctor may offer you some pain medication, which you should consider if your discomfort is significant.

If you had a long labor, did a lot of pushing, and slept only a little the night before, don't be surprised if you also find yourself with a whopper of a headache in the first few hours after birth. Additionally, about 1 in every 100 women who have an epidural—a locally administered labor anesthesia—develop what is known as a spinal headache. Most often fluids and bed rest will help. In rare instances doctors may draw blood from your arm and introduce it into your spinal canal (called a "blood patch") to seal off leakages of spinal fluid that may be contributing to your head pain.

You can also expect to feel a bit woozy and light-headed the first few times you get out of bed. This is also normal, particularly if you had an epidural or any pain medication during delivery.

THE FIRST SIX DAYS: WHAT YOU NEED TO KNOW

The overwhelming fatigue you felt after birth will likely lift after a few hours of rest, but you can expect to feel extremely tired for about the first seven days following your baby's birth. Since feeding your new baby can play havoc with any sleep schedule, you may be getting little rest at night, so you can quickly begin to feel overwhelmed and desperately sleepy. By the seventh or eighth day, the extreme fatigue should be lifting, though you may still feel somewhat tired, particularly during the day. Remember, however, if you lost a lot of blood and/or fluids during delivery, it may take you a few extra days or even weeks before you begin to approach the strength you had before birth.

Within the first seventy-two hours after having your baby, your breasts rapidly produce a great abundance of milk. Simultaneously, blood vessels fill to capacity, causing surrounding breast tissue to swell. The problem, known as engorgement, can be very painful, with tenderness extending all the way into your armpits. Your breasts may feel lumpy as well, and painful to the touch. Fortunately, as soon as your milk is expressed on a regular basis, these problems will quickly resolve.

If you are not breast-feeding, the pain can continue until your milk supply begins to dry—a week or more. During this time, avoid emptying your breasts for relief. While doing so may help temporarily, it will also signal your body to make more milk, which will prolong the pain and the drying process. Also avoid nipple stimulation or warm water on your breasts, both of which encourage milk production. Wearing a support bra or binding your breasts can help ease the pain. Ice packs can also help speed the drying process.

YOUR BODY: WHAT TO EXPECT

Your lochia, or bloody vaginal discharge, will also continue throughout the first week, and may even increase slightly as you return home from the hospital and spend more time on your feet. This increase should last just a few hours and then taper off. Bleeding should continue to decrease so that by week's end it resembles a light menstrual flow, which can continue for several more weeks.

You may also experience "after pains," or uterine contractions, for several days following delivery—a signal that your uterus is shrinking back to its original, prepregnancy size. But unless your pain is severe, doctors say that you should make every effort *not* to remain in bed when you return home. The more you can walk around, the better your circulation and your overall health will be.

You may also notice that you are continuing to experience pressure on your bladder, which in turn can create a constant urge to urinate, as well as make holding urine more difficult. This problem will correct it-self in time, but to speed things up, you may want to begin doing Kegel exercises (see Chapter 5), which you can start as soon as your V zone is healed and not causing you any significant pain.

Most of the achiness you felt after delivery should begin to diminish a few days after birth, except for pain related to a C-section or an epi-siotomy. In this case, you may continue to experience varying levels of discomfort for several more weeks, so don't expect the first six days to bring you any dramatic relief. If you do experience *significant* pain, talk to your doctor about the use of Tylenol (acetaminophen) to aid in your recovery.

THE FIRST SIX WEEKS: WHAT YOU NEED TO KNOW

As you get used to your new baby, and as your new baby adjusts to his or her new world, the fatigue you felt the first week or two after delivery should gradually disappear and be replaced by an increasing sense of en-ergy. By week four you should also be somewhat adjusted to your new sleep schedule. If you are not, be sure to mention this to your doctor dur-ing your first postpartum checkup, which should be about six weeks after delivery.

Although most of your uterine contractions and "after pains" should be gone within the first couple of weeks, your uterus may not assume its normal, prepregnancy shape and size for up to seven weeks. That means you may still feel some bloating or discomfort, and your stomach may re-main quite large. While many women expect to emerge from childbirth with their tummies flat, this virtually never happens. Stretch marks, how-ever, should begin to fade into a soft silvery hue, and varicose veins may also begin to grow lighter and less noticeable.

If you had an episiotomy, it could take the first six weeks—or longer—to fully heal. You can also continue to experience some perineum pain if your V zone was stretched or torn during delivery.

Constipation may be a temporary problem for you now, either be-cause your incision causes bowel movements to be painful, or simply because of normal postpartum changes. If this is the case, don't strain, particularly if you suffered with hemorrhoids during pregnancy. Instead, talk to your doctor about a stool softener, and add more fluids and fiber to your diet.

You may also find that you are continuing to battle incontinence during these first six weeks. As your uterus begins to shrink back to its original size and your pelvic organs and abdomen begin to heal, you should see a gradual improvement. Again, Kegel exercises can help, but so can simply waiting it out; often postpartum incontinence corrects itself.

Because you carry lots of extra water in the weeks following delivery, don't be surprised if you find yourself sweating more than usual. You may even experience some "hot flashes" as hormone levels begin to stabilize.

YOUR BREASTS, SKIN, AND HAIR: WHAT TO EXPECT

If you are breast-feeding, then anytime during the first six weeks you may develop sore, cracked nipples that burn, along with burning, throbbing, or shooting pains in your breasts. Often this is the result of poor "latching"—meaning your baby is not connecting properly to your breast during feeding. If your newborn cries a lot and exhibits other signs of hunger, latching on may be the problem, so talk to your doctor or a lactation counselor. To help ease nipple pain, try creams such as Belli Cosmetics Pure Comfort Nursing Cream, a pharmaceutical-grade lanolin balm that both soothes and heals; PureLan 100 Nipple Lotion by Medela, a 100 percent pure lanolin product; Comforting Nipple Salve by Bella Mamma, a blend of shea butter, olive oil, jojoba oil, plus vitamins E and A; or Lansinoh, a high-grade lanolin cream, samples of which are often available in many hospitals. (See the Resource Center.) Or, after feeding, simply let some breast milk linger on your nipples and air dry. Wash your nipples only once daily with plain water, avoiding all soaps, gels, and washes.

About 5 percent of new moms with latching problems also develop a breast infection known as mastitis. This will cause your breasts to become painful and develop hot, red streaks. You can run a fever of 101 degrees or more and have flulike aches and pains. Although it's not dangerous to breast-feed with mastitis, you will need an antibiotic to clear up the infection, so make certain to call your doctor.

If you are breast-feeding, you can also expect the increased size, shape, and fullness of your breasts to remain for at least several months, followed by a slow decrease in size. If you are not breast-feeding, your breasts will begin looking and feeling more like they did prior to pregnancy within the first six weeks.

Your skin will also begin a series of changes after delivery, beginning with your pregnancy mask, which will start to fade. So will the linea nigra, or "line of pregnancy," on your tummy. However, at least some of the complexion problems you may have experienced when you first got pregnant, such as breakouts or an increase in oiliness, may be back. Since it could take up to two months or more for hormone levels to stabilize after pregnancy, expect anything from temporary acne flare-ups to bouts of dry skin—or a combination of both. Many of the same pampering routines found earlier in this book can do double duty and work well after baby is born.

You may also begin to notice a considerable hair loss or extreme problems styling your hair. This can begin as soon as one month after giving birth or as late as three or four months after your baby is born. Why does it occur? Pregnancy hormones force a change in the natural cycle of hair growth. So, while you are pregnant, hair that normally would be shed on a regular basis stays put; this is one reason why you may appear to have so much more hair during pregnancy.

After delivery, however, hormones shift again and send another message to your hair follicles—one that stimulates all those extra hairs you kept during pregnancy to begin shedding. As a result, it can seem that you're losing handfuls of hair, but in reality you should be experiencing a diffuse shedding occurring evenly throughout your head. You should not end up with any less hair than you had before you were pregnant, and the shedding process should stop eight to ten weeks from the time it starts.

If, however, hair loss is extensive—if you see significant bald spots or if hair is coming out in chunks and clumps—you could be suffering from a form of pregnancy-related thyroid disorder. To know for sure, talk to your doctor about a blood test for thyroid-stimulating hormone (TSH). For more information, see "An Expert's Opinion on Postpartum Fatigue" later in this chapter.

TWELVE REASONS TO CALL YOUR DOCTOR AFTER YOUR BABY IS BORN

According to childbirth expert and obstetrician Dr. Curtis Glade, there are a number of warning signs you should be aware of following delivery, particularly in the first six days after giving birth. While any of these problems can occur anytime during your recovery period, if they occur at all, they are most likely to happen during the first week. Keep an eye out for these symptoms and call your doctor right away if they appear.

- ✓ A temperature of 101 degrees or more (after the first twenty-four hours)

- ✓ Painful, hot, swollen, or red breasts

- ✓ Chills

- ✓ Loss of appetite

- ✓ Pain in the lower abdomen or lower back, or pain, tenderness, or swelling in the lower leg

- ✓ Severe constipation

- ✓ Severe pain in the vagina or perineum

- ✓ Heavy bleeding or sudden increase in bleeding—soaking more than two pads in thirty minutes

- ✓ Vaginal discharge with a strong, foul odor

- ✓ Feelings of extreme sadness, fear, anger, depression, or anxiety

- ✓ Overwhelming fatigue that keeps you from caring for yourself or your baby

- ✓ Extreme negative feelings toward your baby or feelings that you might harm your baby

An Expert's Opinion on

POSTPARTUM FATIGUE

While you can expect some fatigue to linger for the first few weeks after giving birth, when it goes on too long, another problem may be at work. For some, it's a sign of postpartum depression—which you'll learn more about in a few moments. But for up to 15 percent of new moms, fatigue is an indication of a pregnancy-related thyroid disorder. The condition, called postpartum thyroiditis, develops when pregnancy causes your immune system to go slightly awry and attack your thyroid.

"This is an autoimmune reaction, which initially can cause you to feel nervous, with lots of excess energy, and sometimes feelings of fear or anxiety, usually within the first month or two after giving birth," says Dr. Loren Wisner-Greene, a clinical associate professor of endocrinology at New York University School of Medicine. But within a relatively short time, she says, a sudden drop in thyroid function occurs, leaving you feeling extremely fatigued and less able to cope, symptoms that closely resemble those of postpartum depression.

"Because so many of the symptoms of thyroid disorder mimic either those of postpartum depression or even those of ordinary postpartum recovery—such as hair loss or fatigue—many doctors overlook this problem," says Dr. Wisner-Greene. And while a simple blood test that measures levels of thyroid-stimulating hormone, or TSH, can quickly and easily verify a thyroid disorder, too often, she says, women aren't offered the test at their six-week checkup.

"It should be a routine part of the postpartum six-week exam—and

Finally, be aware that most new moms feel some sense of "baby blues" as well as hormone-mediated ups and downs during the first six weeks of recovery. However, these feelings should begin lifting by around the fourth or fifth week after delivery. If they don't, discuss this with your doctor during your first postpartum visit. (See "When the Baby Blues Won't Go Away: What to Do" later in this chapter.)

if your doctor doesn't recommend it, you should bring it up, particularly if you are feeling extremely fatigued and even somewhat depressed," says Wisner-Greene.

For the most part, "normal" postpartum fatigue gradually *lifts*. Each day you feel less tired, more energetic, and more in tune with your body and your baby. By the third week you should feel a substantial decrease in your tiredness and more in control of your immediate surroundings and your life.

If, however, you still feel as overwhelmed by the end of week two or three as you did the day after delivery, or if you feel worse as the days go by, contact your doctor as soon as possible and ask about the thyroid test.

Should a problem be detected, one of several medications—safe to take while breast-feeding—can control symptoms. Or your doctor may choose to take a wait-and-see approach, since often thyroid function reverts to normal on its own. It is important, however, that your health is monitored during this waiting period to ensure that you are recovering.

Signs of an Overactive Thyroid (Hyperthyroidism): Heat intolerance; increased appetite; weight loss; heart rate greater than 100 beats per minute; heart palpitations (feeling your heart race or skip a beat); insomnia; tremors.

Signs of an Underactive Thyroid (Hypothyroidism): Cold intolerance; decreased appetite; constipation; inability to lose weight or weight gain; dry skin; depression; fatigue; hair loss.

Getting Your Body Back in Shape: Where to Begin

If you are like many women, from almost the moment you give birth you'll be fantasizing about getting back into that little black cocktail dress or gray pinstripe pantsuit, or maybe even your favorite bikini. At the same time, don't be too surprised if you are also feeling so totally overwhelmed with your new life and your new baby that getting back into your exercise routine and losing that extra weight seem like the impossible dream.

In either case, the decision about when to begin the task of slimming down and shaping up is totally up to you. While in the past doctors routinely recommended that all pregnant women wait at least six weeks after giving birth before even attempting any exercise, this is no longer true. The latest recommendations by the American College of Obstetricians and Gynecologists is to let your personal health be your guide. They say it's okay to begin exercising much sooner than in the past, as long as your body is up to the task.

At the same time, it's important that you don't feel pressure to begin working out or dieting before you are really ready. If your new baby is consuming all your time, enjoy it, and don't worry about dieting or exercising just yet. There certainly will be plenty of time to do that in the future.

Likewise, don't be overly influenced by the publicity surrounding Hollywood's new brigade of "Yummy Mommies"—gorgeous, glamorous new-mom superstars such as Cindy Crawford, Sarah Jessica Parker, Catherine Zeta-Jones, Liz Hurley, Brooke Shields, Julianne Moore, Kelly Ripa, Claudia Schiffer, Jennifer Connelly, and Kate Moss—to name a few! In the spotlight throughout their pregnancies, and particularly shortly after giving birth, their natural good looks combined with an ability to get their bodies back in what seems like moments after delivery, have set the bar high for pregnancy recovery.

Certainly, they make great role models for today's "Hot Mamma," particularly by showing us just how spectacular a mom, and particularly a new mom, can look. Still, don't let their fast recoveries intimidate you, or push you into trying to achieve a nearly impossible goal. Remember, most of these women have unlimited time and money to spend on themselves. Most also have full- or part-time child care, household help, cooks, nutritionists, personal trainers, and personal assistants at their disposal, not to mention hairdressers, make-up artists, and stylists to help out. Indeed, it's far easier to get to that Pilates class three times a week and eat those low-fat gourmet meals when you're not running around emptying poop pails, cleaning spit-up, washing dirty clothes, grocery shopping, and cooking! Not to mention tending to your new little one—and maybe one or two others in tow!

The bottom line: When it comes to finding a role model for post-natal recovery, do emulate their sassy Hollywood style and follow their drop-dead-gorgeous examples. But don't set your recovery goals so impossibly high that you end up driving yourself too hard, particularly in the days and weeks immediately following delivery. Doing so could contribute to a postpartum depression, or at least dampen your otherwise joyous spirits with some unnecessary pressures.

If, however, you *are* raring to get your old self back sooner rather than later, there are some sane and sensible ways to do just that.

Your Postpregnancy Workouts: What's Safe, What's Not

Generally speaking, doctors say it's safest to begin your early postpreg-nancy fitness regimen with the same workout you were doing in the very last stages of your pregnancy. This probably included simple movements, like modified sit-ups and stretches. Weather permitting, walking is always a good choice, particularly if you can take your baby along in a carriage or a front-held knapsack.

If your episiotomy is not yet healed or if you are experiencing any pain in this area, it's probably not a good idea to do any floor exercises. And, if working out brings on muscle pain or nausea, or if your bloody discharge increases or begins again, then you are doing too much too soon.

While it's also not a great idea to concentrate on dieting too soon af-ter birth, if, in fact, you are trying to watch your weight, never go for more than a one-pound loss per week—and this includes diet and exercise combined. Losing too much weight too quickly can contribute to fatigue and may increase your risk of postpartum depression. Because your body needs time to restore the nutritional balance that was disrupted by preg-nancy and delivery, doctors continue to suggest that strict dieting be avoided for at least the first few months after childbirth. This is particu-larly important if you are nursing, since you are going to need the extra nutrition and, possibly, additional calories.

As to the shape of your tummy, you should expect to see your "preg-nancy pouch" for at least several weeks after delivery. While some women can get back those rock-hard abs and flat tummy shortly after birth, this is rare. In fact, the speed at which you get your body back depends on what your normal weight was before pregnancy, how much weight you gained, as well as your activity level both before and during pregnancy. Studies show that limiting weight gain to no more than thirty pounds and exercising regularly while you are pregnant can make it easier to return to your preconception weight.

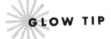

GLOW TIP

Losing Your Baby Fat

During pregnancy, women typically store fat in their lower abdomen and upper thighs. It's normal for these areas to retain fat after giving birth. The best way to get rid of it is to exercise regularly, which will decrease overall fat. Breast-feeding also helps reduce this sex-specific fat because your body burns a greater amount of energy to create breast milk. *Be patient.* It took nine months to gain the weight that significantly changed your body. Expect it to take at least six to nine months to reverse those changes. Try to relax and enjoy this special time with your child.

Tamilee Webb, *Buns of Steel*

Sex and the Afterglow:
What You Need to Know

In the past, most doctors routinely recommended no sex for six weeks—giving women an automatic time frame in which they didn't even have to think about intimate relations, much less have them. Today, however, the "rules" are more liberal, with many physicians suggesting that as long as there was no episiotomy and no birthing complications, sexual activity, including intercourse, can begin as soon as bleeding stops, which for many women occurs in just two to three weeks.

Don't be surprised, however, if the idea of resuming intimate rela-

IS YOUR BELLY READY FOR EXERCISE?
HOW TO TELL

During pregnancy you may have developed something called diastasis of the rectus—meaning that your stomach muscles (the *recti abdominis)* pulled apart slightly, allowing your baby more room to grow. After delivery, these muscles come back together—but exercising too soon could keep this from happening.

To tell if your tummy is ready for exercise, try this simple test: Lie on your back with your knees bent. Place the palm of your left hand just over your navel. Take a deep breath and, as you begin to exhale, lift your head, neck, and shoulders off the floor (as if you were starting to do a sit-up). At the same time, slide your right hand up your thigh, reaching toward your knee (again as if you were going to do a sit-up). Hold this position for a few seconds—long enough for your left hand (just over your navel) to touch your stomach muscles and see if you can feel a gap between the left and right sides of your belly. If that gap is wider than the width of three fingers, it means your stomach muscles have not yet come back together, so strenuous abdominal exercises are not a good idea. Once the space between your muscles narrows to one finger in width, you are ready for crunches or other advanced abdominal exercises. However, don't jump into a heavy workout right away. To minimize the risk of damage to your stomach muscles, start slowly and build up to a more strenuous workout gradually, as you recover. Of course, if you had a cesarean section delivery, all stomach exercises are off limits until your incision is fully healed and your doctor gives you the okay to begin working out.

tions is *not* on the top of your list for quite some time after baby is born. A number of medical studies now show that a woman's reluctance to have sex after pregnancy, as well as the incidence of postpartum V zone pain, is more widespread than previously thought. In research published in 1999 in the *Journal of Reproductive Medicine,* a group of Oregon doctors found that nearly six months after giving birth, up to 47 percent of the women in their study were still having pain during sex, with up to one-third suf-

Real Life

BREAST-FEEDING AND
POSTPREGNANCY WEIGHT LOSS

Q: A friend told me that breast-feeding helps you lose weight after pregnancy. Is this true? I think it's the opposite—that all the extra calories you need for breast-feeding make you fatter longer. Who is right?

A: Listen to your girlfriend, girlfriend, because in the short run it's true, breast-feeding *can* help you lose weight. Studies show that making milk burns calories, so weight seems to drop off faster. Breast-feeding also causes the release of the hormone oxytocin, which, in turn, causes your uterus to contract and shrink back to its original size, which can make your tummy look better.

In the long run, however, many moms say they have problems losing the last five or ten pounds until they stop breast-feeding. Some doctors believe the body holds on to these extra fat stores to help ensure enough nutritional support to continue to make milk. In addition, expect your breasts to be larger than they were before pregnancy; generally they will stay that way until you finish nursing.

fering severe sexual dysfunction. For nearly half of the women, some degree of pelvic and perineal tenderness lasted up to one year. Likewise, research published in the *American Journal of Obstetrics and Gynecology* in 2001 revealed that women who suffer severe perineal trauma during birth are up to 270 times more likely to experience extreme pain during sex, even months after their baby is born. This same study also revealed that women who breast-feed are up to four times more likely to experience painful sex for up to six months after giving birth—a phenomenon also cited in the Oregon study.

Even if you had a simple, easy birth, sex *still* may be the last thing on your mind. One reason is that for most women, sexual desire is intimately tied to hormonal activity. So, frequently, desire won't return until your menstrual cycle is back on track, which can take two months or more.

In terms of those extra breast-feeding calories—in the first few months after delivery, your body has almost everything it needs to produce enough milk. But because making milk burns about 300 to 500 calories a day, in the past, doctors routinely advised women to add that same number of calories to what they might normally eat to maintain their weight.

Today, however, that line of thinking has somewhat changed. Many doctors now believe that unless you are *very* underweight, what you and your baby really need is good nutrition and a well-balanced diet, and not necessarily more calories. In fact, as long as you eat nutritiously—lots of fresh fruits, vegetables, and whole grains, as well as low-fat dairy products and adequate protein—then what you burn making milk *can* help you lose those extra pounds faster and more easily.

If, however, you are losing more than one pound per week, or you reach your prepregnancy weight and continue to lose, then you should definitely increase your caloric intake and maintain a higher calorie diet until you have finished breast-feeding.

Additionally, depending on the circumstances under which you became pregnant—particularly if it was a surprise—as well as how you feel about being a mother and how your partner and your family are reacting to the birth, you may feel you want to avoid sex or even have somewhat of a temporary aversion to making love after your baby is born.

However, as your hormones come back to normal, and you become more comfortable with your baby and your role as a mother, these feelings of avoidance should pass. If they continue, and particularly if you want to make love but find that you can't, talk to your doctor about medical treatments and the possibility of counseling to help you get your intimate life back on track.

It's also important to remember that, for many women, the sheer exhaustion of caring for a newborn will leave little time, or desire, for sex. In at least some instances, cuddling, touching, and holding your newborn all day long, particularly if you are nursing, may leave you feeling "all touched out" and in no mood for physical contact of any kind by day's end.

Most important is to realize that no two women are alike, so no two recovery periods will be the same. While some women who receive an episiotomy or other lacerations may heal fully within two to four weeks after birth, and may begin enjoying sex right away, others who had only minimal incisions may continue to feel some pain and discomfort for three to five months after delivery. The same is true for every other factor related to sex after pregnancy, including not only hormonal fluctuations, but also emotional factors linked to readiness.

The bottom line: You are on your own personal timetable, so don't pressure yourself to resume intimate relations before you are physically or emotionally ready.

Whenever you do feel the time is right to begin making love, remember, you *can* get pregnant again—sometimes sooner than you realize. While breast-feeding does decrease your chances for conceiving, it's not a guarantee, so talk to your doctor about which method of birth control might be best for you at this time. If you can't or don't want to use the Pill, and if a diaphragm would not be comfortable or convenient, talk to your partner about using condoms, at least for a short time. Be aware, however, that spermacides or sometimes condoms themselves may cause vaginal tissue that is still a bit delicate to become inflamed. If this happens, abstain from sex until you are fully healed.

Even if, with all things considered, you feel that your sex life may *never* be the same again, there are things that you can do to help encourage a gradual return to intimacy and in some instances even overcome some obstacles standing in your way. What follows are some suggestions that noted experts say can help put your intimate life back on track.

Seven Ways to Put Sex Back in Your Life

1. **Never Underestimate the Power of a Good Lubricant!** Reduced levels of estrogen following childbirth, combined with increases in the hormones prolactin and oxytocin, can leave your V zone feeling dry and irritated, particularly if you are breast-feeding. This can not only make intercourse painful, it can even diminish desire. To overcome both problems, choose a water-based lubricant (most child-

birth experts recommend Astroglide, K-Y Brand Lubricating Jelly, or Liquid Silk) and begin using it regularly, even when you aren't planning an intimate encounter.

2. **Don't Try to "Switch Gears" from Mom to Lover Too Soon.** Perhaps nothing takes away sexual desire more than changing dirty diapers and burping Baby Snooks! Don't try to go from nursery to the love bed without taking a pause to regroup. To break the cycle of mommydom, spend a little time with your mate—even just ten minutes sipping a glass of wine or talking—before attempting to become intimate.

3. **Don't Confuse Sex with Affection.** Just because you may not feel ready to have intercourse, don't overlook the power of affectionate behavior to encourage a closer bond between you and your partner. Studies show that touching in a warm affectionate way—holding hands or cuddling—can influence hormones that affect sexual desire. You may be surprised to see how quickly you can go from cuddling to caressing to intercourse.

4. **Think Outside the Bed.** Don't limit intimate encounters to the bedroom or to the evening hours. If you're just too pooped to pop by the end of the day, put a little spontaneity into your romantic life and consider being intimate at different times and perhaps in different rooms of your home. Also, don't feel inhibited about making love with baby around; it's perfectly okay. In fact, if you're a nervous mom, always listening for baby's cries, having your newborn in the same room can help you relax and enjoy your partner more.

5. **Embrace Change.** Accept the fact that intercourse may feel a little uncomfortable the first few times. That doesn't mean it should cause intense or even significant pain. But if your vagina simply feels a little "tight" or "sore," recognize that this will likely pass after a few encounters. On the opposite end of the spectrum, a temporary decrease in the tone of your perineal muscles could mean there is less friction during intercourse, which could make orgasms less intense and harder to achieve. The Kegel exercises described

earlier can help. It's also important to realize that your sexual encounters are going to feel different as you and your partner approach lovemaking a little more cautiously than before. This too is normal and will soon pass as you once again get used to each other, and to making love.

6. **Keep the Lines of Communication Open.** Make certain your partner knows and fully understands what you are feeling and why. Encourage your mate to discuss his feelings about your current sex life, and make certain that he knows his attractiveness has not faded. While you'll both be exhausted from the new-baby schedule, it's imperative that you find at least one hour, once or twice a week, to spend together—talking, holding hands, watching a movie, or having a meal. Try not to talk about baby during this time; concentrate on being together.

Also be aware that, in rare circumstances, your mate may find it more difficult than you to return to your former intimate life. Some men may be temporarily turned off by making love to a "mother" (they are putting you in the same category as their own mom), and some may have been so traumatized by watching the birth of their child that they are petrified that you will get pregnant again. In the first scenario, you can break the "mom" complex by making extra sure to spend time together *without* your new baby— even if it's just the two of you alone in the next room. Make a promise to talk just about each other, and try, at least mentally, to turn back the clock to your prepregnancy days. Play favorite songs or arrange to do something romantic together that you did before pregnancy—anything to jar his thinking in a different direction can help. In most instances his fears will pass and the sexual feelings he had for you will quickly return.

In cases in which his emotional reaction to birth trauma is keeping you apart, birth control can play a major role in helping to ease his fears. Being certain you won't get pregnant again—at least not right now—may help ease whatever fears he is harboring from the birthing experience. In addition, it's true that time heals all wounds—and like any other traumatic event in your lives, eventually you will both forget any of the trauma associated with giving birth, as these feelings gradually are replaced with the joy of watching your baby develop and grow.

7. **Talk to Your Doctor.** If sex continues to be painful, and lubricants don't help, don't hesitate to talk to your doctor about whatever difficulties you are experiencing. Sometimes there are medical reasons behind your problems, and treatments can help. On occasion there may even be a delivery-related physical condition influencing your ability to enjoy sex—such as tight sutures that can make intercourse painful. If this is the case, your doctor can instruct you on how to slowly dilate your vagina until sex becomes more comfortable.

Giving Birth and Your Emotions: Some Important News

Most women are overjoyed to become mothers—each and every time it occurs. Moreover, the thrill of holding, feeding, and cuddling your *first* child for the *first* time can be an experience second to none. But even if you are completely enthralled with motherhood, don't be surprised if your postpartum recovery also includes a few emotions you were not expecting—including fear, sadness, self-doubt, anxiety, irritability, even feelings of anger toward your baby. According to experts from the American College of Obstetricians and Gynecologists, at least some form of emotional upset affects up to 80 percent of all new mothers. Collectively called the "baby blues," these symptoms are so common that in many medical circles they are considered a "normal" part of pregnancy.

You should also know that the baby blues normally set in quickly—you could start feeling symptoms a day or two after delivery. These feelings are driven by the dramatic changes in hormone levels, which plummet just after giving birth. If you suffered with premenstrual syndrome (PMS) prior to getting pregnant, you may respond to these changes more dramatically now. You can even expect some mood swings and other symptoms similar to what you experienced prior to each menstrual cycle.

But raging hormones alone are not the whole problem. A lack of sleep as well as physical problems related to your recovery can also contribute to these "down" feelings. Emotional upset can seem worse if your partner or family were not supportive of your pregnancy or of your new baby.

For most women, the worst of these up-and-down feelings will peak between the fifth and seventh day following delivery, and often resolve completely within seventy-two hours. While you may continue to feel sensitive or a little overemotional for a while, over the course of the next five weeks you will continue to feel a little better each day, until you are once again feeling yourself.

When the Baby Blues Won't Go Away: What to Do

While most women—even those with dramatic cases of the baby blues—feel much better by the end of their second postpartum week, for some, emotional upset can continue unabated for weeks. For still others, the postpartum period can seem void of any dramatic feelings—only to be followed by an upswing in emotions, particularly depression, setting in two or three months *after* giving birth.

In both instances, the problem is known as postpartum depression. Characterized as an overwhelming and increasing sense of sadness that builds over time, according to the American College of Obstetricians and Gynecologists, postpartum depression affects up to 20 percent of all new mothers. At its worst, a woman can feel totally overwhelmed with sadness and unable to care for herself or her baby. According to Dr. Kathryn Leopold, assistant professor of obstetrics and gynecology at Albany Medical College, most women who develop postpartum depression can still be experiencing symptoms six months after birth. If left untreated, 25 percent will still be suffering from depression a year after their baby is born.

POSTPARTUM DEPRESSION: ARE YOU AT RISK?

Although doctors aren't sure why some women fall prey to this problem while others do not, evidence points to extremes in hormonal activity, combined with other dramatic physical and lifestyle changes occurring in the weeks following delivery. Some research also shows that genetics may play a role as well. In much the same way that some women appear to be more susceptible to mood swings or other symptoms during their monthly menstrual cycle, so too can some women be genetically sensitive to the physiological changes that occur in the body following the birth of a child.

A study conducted by researcher Elizabeth Corwin, assistant professor at the Penn State School of Nursing, offers another theory: that fatigue may, in fact, play the biggest role of all. In studies presented in 2002 at the Scientific Session of the Eastern Nursing Research Society in University Park, Pennsylvania, Corwin offered important new evidence that fatigue may actually be the red alert that identifies women at greatest risk for postpartum depression.

Certainly, all women feel tired following childbirth and for several weeks afterward. But as the study discovered, in most women there is a curve, with the fatigue gradually lessening over time. However, in women who are prone to depression, that curve is not seen, and fatigue takes on a different pattern. Instead of gradually reducing, it continues, so much so that a woman can feel as tired, or even more tired, on day fourteen as she felt on day seven, which should normally not be the case after giving birth. It was no surprise when researchers discovered that those women who continued to experience extreme, unrelenting fatigue two weeks after giving birth were also at highest risk for developing postpartum depression.

The key realization here: If your fatigue continues and does not lift within two weeks after childbirth, or if your fatigue increases and actually grows worse over time, you may be at increased risk for postpartum depression—and it's important that intervention take place as soon as possible.

For Kathryn Lee, professor of nursing at the University of California at San Francisco, postpartum depression is a classic representation of sleep deprivation. "It's not a mental, psychotic breakdown, it's really that [these women] are totally sleep-deprived," reported Lee.

Although sometimes the baby blues can progress to full-blown postpartum depression, women who suffer postpartum depression do not usually progress to the more serious postpartum psychosis—a severe form of depression that completely alters a woman's ability to think rationally about her children or her life. Affecting only a very small number of women, this disorder is completely different and not something that most women need to worry about.

What makes all this new research so important, however, is that using fatigue as a guide, you and your doctor may be able to spot your risk for postpartum depression and intervene before problems get out of hand. You can, for example, arrange to have a family member or a day nanny take care of your new baby for a few hours every day while you grab some much-needed sleep. This strategy is extremely important if feelings of fatigue or sadness are not lifting. Also important: Talk to your doctor about how you feel, including your fears and anxieties.

If you are diagnosed with postpartum depression, there are medications, such as antidepressants or sometimes hormonal therapy, that can help. Most often you will begin to feel better in several weeks, and your depression may lift completely within a few short months. Be certain, however, that you receive a full checkup, including a blood test to measure thyroid function, before you begin any treatment for depression.

Babying Mom: A Few Final Words

When I began researching and writing this book, my intention was to offer you a simple, easy guide to caring for yourself and your needs during pregnancy. And it is my hope that the information I have provided will help you do just that. But in the process of writing these chapters, I began to realize that while pedicures and foot massages, new hairdos and home spas can help you cope with some of your pregnancy woes, what really affects the way you feel the most is maintaining a calm, relaxed, and positive *attitude* about becoming a mom.

Most of you probably already feel this way—perhaps this was the reason you decided to get pregnant at this time in your life. But if, by chance, you are feeling a little confused, anxious, or even fearful about how the months ahead may unfold, I hope you will take some measure of comfort in knowing that pregnancy and childbirth are not illnesses, but rather one of nature's most glorious miracles, and a sign that you are a healthy, vibrant woman.

So while there may be morning sickness and contractions, backaches, foot aches, and enough red and blue stretch marks to turn your tummy into a road map, never forget that one of the main reasons we are all here on this earth is lying just inside your belly, waiting patiently for all the love and affection you can muster. Enjoy every moment of your pregnancy, and revel in the fact that you are part of the miracle that is making the world go round.

I wish good health and happiness, now and in the future, for you, your baby, and your family. Thank you for allowing me to share in what I know will be among the happiest and most memorable times of your life.

The Resource Center

Cosmetics, Skin Care, Bath, and Beauty Products

Adrienne Arpel's Industrial
Concealer
800-284-3100
www.hsn.com

Almost Natural Nail Polish Remover
www.janetbond.com/naturalpolish
remover.htm

Astroglide
866-TRY-ASTRO (free samples!)
www.astroglide.com

Aura Cacia Cocoa Butter
800-425-3115
www.smartbomb.com

Aveeno Itch Relief with Natural
Colloidal Oatmeal
877-298-2525
www.drugstore.com

Avon's Anew All-in-One Perfecting
Lotion, Perfecting Creme
800-500-AVON
www.avon.com

Belli Cosmetics
425-313-5878
www.bellicosmetics.com

Bobbi Brown
www.bobbibrown.com

Burt's Bees Dusting Powder
www.burtsbees.com

California Baby
877-576-2825
www.californiababy.com

Camouflage Dermacolor
800-MakeUp4
www.laurageller.com

Color Enhancing Shampoo
877-LaLucci
www.susanlucci.com

Daily Facials by Oil of Olay
800-241-2701
www.oilofolay.com

Depends
www.walgreens.com

Dermablend QUICK Fix Kit, Duo
Correction
877-900-6700
www.dermablend.com

Dr. Hauschka
800-247-9907
www.drhauschka.com

Evian Face Mister
877-SEPHORA
www.sephora.com

Go Natural Non-Toxic Nail Polish
www.hypoallergenic-nail-polish.com

Gynecort Anti-Itch
800-431-2610
www.vagisil.com

Johnson and Johnson Cornstarch
Baby Powder
866-565-2229
www.johnsonsbaby.com/pro_
powder.asp

K-Y Personal Lubricant Jelly
www.drugstore.com

Laura Geller Cosmetics
800-MakeUp4
www.laurageller.com

L'Occitane
888-623-2880
www.loccitane.com

Magia Bella
800-871-9954
www.magiabella.com

Medela Cosmetics
800-435-8316
www.medela.com

Michael Marons Everything Powder
800-345-1515
www.qvc.com Item #A64970

Neutrogena
800-582-4048
www.neutrogena.com

Orjene
800-88 ORJENE
www.orjene.com

Peel Off Polish
www.bewellstaywell.com/nail_care.htm

Poise
www.poise.com

Ponds Age Defying Lotion for
Delicate Skin
800-743-8640
www.ponds.com

Preggie Pops
866-PREGGIE
www.preggiepops.com

Principal Secret Exfoliating Scrub
800-345-1515
www.qvc.com Item #A8128

Sante Hypoallergenic Nail Polish
www.saffron.com

Sephora
877-SEPHORA
www.sephora.com

Serenity Music
800-869-1684
www.SerenityMusic.com/guided.html

Shea Butter, Avocado and Lemon by
Perlier
800-284-3100
www.hsn.com

SilkenSecret
866-TRY-ASTRO
www.astroglide.com

Slippery Stuff
877-542-3688
www.Wallace-medical.com

Smashbox Cosmetics
800-763-1361
www.smashbox.com

Stiefel Sarna Anti Itch Lotion
888-371-SKIN
www.skinstore.com

St. Ives Gentle Apricot Facial
Scrub
www.stives.com

Tina Cassaday's Salon
310-276-6194
www.hairbyt.com

Tom's of Maine
800-FOR-TOMS (800–367–8667)
www.tomsofmaine.com

Vagisil Deodorant Powder, Vagisil
Anti Itch Creme
800-431-2610
www.vagisil.com

Fashion Passions

Anna Cris Maternity Wear
800–281–2662
www.annacris.com

A Pea in the Pod (Nationwide)
800-273-2763
www.apeainthepod.com
Where the celebs shop for maternity
wear! Designer looks; contemporary
styles; glamour pregnancy wear; career
looks; sexy intimate wear; accessories.

Babystyle
877-Estyles (378-9537)
www.babystyle.com
Another top celebrity maternity site.
Find fashion and beauty advice from
stars like Cindy Crawford, Josie
Bissett, Sarah Jessica Parker, and
more, plus a wide selection of
everyday-to-glam maternity wear,
baby goods, skin care, and more.

Country Dutchess Fashion
Jewely and Accessories
www.countrydutchess.com

Gap Maternity (Nationwide)
800-GapStyle
www.gap.com
Casual wear, jeans, sweats and all
things Gap for mothers-to-be.

Metro Mom
800-Mom-5830
www.metromom.com
Great casual and career clothes in
sizes from small through extra large.
Tall and petite sizing, as well as
pregnancy wear for Orthodox women
with longer sleeves, longer skirts.

Mimi Maternity (Nationwide)
877–MimiMom (877–646-4666)
www.mimimaternity.com
Young, fun contemporary fashions for
work and play.

Motherhood Stores (Nationwide)
800–4Mom2Be (800–466-6223)
www.motherhood.com
Check out the belly option fit guide
page to find the right type of
maternity clothes for your body.
Features plus size as well as regular-
size maternity wear. Or visit
www.imaternity.com, Motherhood's
bargain outlet.

Old Navy Maternity (Nationwide)
800-OLDNAVY
www.oldnavy.com
Inexpensive but stylish maternity
wear available in stores nationwide or
online.

QVC
800-345-1212
www.QVC.com

ShapeEssentials
www.KathleenKirkwood.com
888-552-8783

Pregnancy Information Websites

www.AmericanBaby.com
www.babycenter.com
www.childbirth.org
www.epregnancy.com
www.fitpregnancy.com
www.ivillage.com
www.parentsplace.com
www.pregnancytoday.com
www.pregnancyweekly.com
www.Storknet.com
www.theVzone.net

Medical Information

MEDICAL ORGANIZATIONS

American Academy of Asthma,
Allergy and Immunology
800-822-2762
www.aaaai.org

American Academy of Dermatology
888-462-DERM
www.aad.org

American Academy of Family
Physicians
www.familydoctor.org

American College of Asthma, Allergy
and Immunology
800-842-7777
www.allergy.mcg.edu

American College of Obstetricians
and Gynecologists (ACOG)
www.acog.org

American College of Radiology
800-ACR-LINE
www.ACR.org

American College of Sports
Medicine
317-637-9200 ext. 138
www.acsm.org

American Council for Headache
Education (ACHE)
856-423-0258
www.achenet.org

American Dietetic Association
800-877-1600
www.eatright.org

American Lung Association
212-315-8700
www.lungusa.org

American Medical Association
312-464-5000
www.ama-assn.org

American Society of Dermatologic
Surgery
847-956-0900
www.aboutskinsurgery.com

American Society of Hypertension
212-696-9099
www.ash-us.org

Center for Science in the Public
Interest
202-332-9110
www.cspinet.org

March of Dimes
800-996-2724
www.Modimes.org

National Association of Pregnancy
Massage Therapists (NAPMT)
888-451-4945
email: NAPMT@Texas.net

National Institute of Relationship
Enhancement
800-4Families
www.nire.org

National Sleep Foundation
202-347-3471
www.sleepfoundation.org

Organization of Teratology
Information Services
866-626-OTIS
www.otispregnancy.org

Royal College of Obstetricians and
Gynecologists
www.rcog.org.uk

SIDS—American SIDS Institute
800-232-SIDS
www.SIDS.org

Society of Behavioral Medicine
608-827-7267
www.sbmweb.org

MEDICAL JOURNALS

Alcoholism: Clinical and Experimental Research
www.alcoholism-cer.com

American Journal of Clinical Nutrition
www.ajcn.org

American Journal of Epidemiology
aje.oupjournals.org

American Journal of Obstetrics and Gynecology
www.us.elsevierhealth.com

British Journal of Obstetrics and Gynecology
www.womenshealth-elsevier.com/doc/journals.html

British Medical Journal
www.bmj.com

Chest
www.chestjournal.org

The Female Patient
www.femalepatient.com

Journal of Allergy and Clinical Immunology
www.us.elsevierhealth.com

Journal of the American Dietetic Association
www.eatright.org/journal

Journal of the American Medical Association
jama.ama-assn.org

Journal of Environmental Health Perspectives
ehpnet1.niehs.nih.gov/docs/all-pubs.html

Journal of Family Planning Perspectives
www.jstor.org/journals/00147354.html

Journal of Obstetrics and Gynecology and Neonatal Nursing
www.nursingcenter.com

Journal of Periodontology
www.perio.org/journal.html

Journal of Psychosomatic Obstetrics and Gynecology
jpog.ispog.org

Journal of Reproductive Medicine
www.reproductivemedicine.com/index2.html

Lancet
thelancet.com

New England Journal of Medicine
www.nejm.org

Obstetrics and Gynecology
www.acog.org

Occupational and Environmental Medicine
www.acoem.org/journal/general.asp

The Physician and Sports Medicine
www.physsportsmed.com

Seminars in Reproductive Medicine
www.thieme.com

Spine
www.spinejournal.com

Government Agencies

Environmental Protection Agency
202-260-2090
www.epa.gov

Food and Drug Administration
888-INFO-FDA
www.fda.gov

Health Care Financing Administration
877-267-2323
www.hcta.gov/medicaid/hipaa/online/00002.asd

National Centers for Disease Control
800-311-3435
www.cdc.gov

National Institute of Child Health and Human Development
www.nichd.nih.gov

National Institute of Occupational Safety and Health
800-35-NIOSH
www.cdc.gov/niosh

National Institutes of Health
301-496-4000
www.nih.gov

National Institutes of Health
National Center for Complementary
and Alternative Medicine
www.nccam.nih.gov

National Institutes of Medicine (of
the National Academy of Sciences)
www.iom.edu

Occupational Safety Health
Association (OSHA)
800-321-6742
www.osha.gov

U.S. Department of Labor
866-4-USA-DOL
www.dol.gov

U.S. Equal Employment
Opportunity Commission
800-669-4000
www.eecoc.gov

U.S. National Research Council
www.nas.edu.nrc

U.S. Pharmacopeia
800-227-8772
www.usp.org

Index

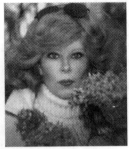

JORGE VERDANI

COLETTE BOUCHEZ is an award-winning medical journalist with more than twenty years' experience. She is the former medical writer for the *New York Daily News*, and the top-selling author of *The V Zone* and co-author of *Getting Pregnant*. Currently a daily medical correspondent for HealthDay News Service/The New York Times Syndicate, her popular consumer health articles appear daily online, as well as in newspapers nationwide and in Europe and Japan. She is a regular contributor to WebMD.com, USAToday.com, ABCNews.com, MSNBC.com, and more than two dozen radio and television news stations nationwide. She lives in New York City.